ULCERATIVE COLITIS COOKBOOK: A DIET PLAN FOR BEGINNERS

A Nutritional Blueprint for Colitis Symptoms Relief, Reducing Inflammation, Improved Gut Health, and Eliminating IBD

Audrey McAllister, MD

Copyright Page

Requests for permission to use or reproduce any part of this publication should be addressed to the publisher in writing. The publisher reserves the right to grant or deny permission at their discretion, taking into consideration factors such as the intended use, nature of the excerpt, and potential impact on the original work.

Unauthorized reproduction or distribution of copyrighted material is a violation of intellectual property rights and may result in legal consequences. Individuals or entities found to be in breach of copyright law may be subject to legal action, including but not limited to injunctions, damages, and legal fees.

It is the responsibility of all users of this publication to familiarize themselves with and abide by copyright laws and regulations. By accessing or using any part of this work, individuals agree to comply with the terms and conditions set forth by the publisher regarding copyright protection and usage rights.

Table of Contents

SECTION 1: WHAT IS ULCERATIVE COLITIS?

Ulcerative colitis, categorized as an inflammatory bowel disease (IBD), inflames and forms ulcers in the digestive tract, particularly affecting the inner lining of the large intestine (colon) and rectum. Symptoms typically progress gradually rather than appearing suddenly. While ulcerative colitis can be debilitating and occasionally lead to severe complications, there is presently no known cure. However, numerous emerging treatments can significantly alleviate symptoms and induce long-term remission.

Ulcerative colitis (UC) constitutes a persistent inflammation of the colon, characterized by `periods of symptom-free remission. Common indications include diarrhea, bloody stools, abdominal cramps, and weight loss. Treatment options encompass medications and, in severe cases, surgical intervention.

UC, a lifelong condition, initiates inflammation and ulcer formation within the colon. It ranks among the prevalent forms of IBD, alongside Crohn's disease, frequently presenting with bloody diarrhea and abdominal discomfort, potentially increasing the frequency of bowel movements.

The disease stems from an immune system malfunction, where ordinarily protective white blood cells erroneously target the colon's lining, mistaking it for foreign invaders such as food, beneficial gut bacteria, or healthy cells. The resultant inflammation and ulcers characterize the condition.

The exact cause of ulcerative colitis remains uncertain, with genetics possibly playing a role, as evidenced by familial clustering of the disease. Other environmental factors may also influence susceptibility.

Factors affecting the likelihood of developing ulcerative colitis include age, with a higher incidence among individuals aged 15 to 30 or over 60, ethnicity, notably in those of Ashkenazi Jewish descent, and familial history, with a potential risk increase of up to 30% if close relatives have the condition.

Do you have a higher likelihood of developing ulcerative colitis?

Ulcerative colitis (UC) is a prevalent condition that impacts a significant portion of the population, with an estimated 1-2 million individuals affected in the United States alone. Surprisingly, it surpasses the prevalence of Crohn's disease, another inflammatory bowel condition. While UC can manifest at any age, it predominantly emerges among individuals under 30 years old, highlighting its prevalence among the younger demographic.

Interestingly, UC does not discriminate based on gender, affecting both males and females, albeit slightly more common in males. Additionally, there are distinct demographic patterns in UC prevalence. Caucasians and individuals of Ashkenazi Jewish descent tend to have a higher incidence of UC compared to Asian, African, and South American populations. Moreover, non-smokers and former smokers are at a higher risk of developing UC, contrasting with the lower incidence observed among current smokers.

Moreover, there's a notable familial component associated with UC. Many patients with UC have relatives who also suffer from inflammatory bowel disease, whether it's UC or Crohn's disease. This familial clustering suggests a genetic predisposition to these conditions, highlighting the importance of understanding family medical history in diagnosing and managing UC.

UC presents itself as a complex and multifaceted condition, with demographic, genetic, and lifestyle factors all playing significant roles in its development and progression. By gaining a deeper understanding of these factors, healthcare professionals can better tailor treatment approaches and support strategies to address the unique needs of individuals living with UC.

Different Types of Ulcerative Colitis

Ulcerative colitis (UC) typically initiates its inflammatory assault in the rectum before gradually advancing upwards along the bowel. The intensity of symptoms hinges on the location of inflammation within the colon, which subsequently allows for the classification of UC into several subtypes:

Proctitis: This subtype exclusively affects the rectum, representing the mildest manifestation of UC. The colon typically functions normally in this scenario, with symptoms primarily revolving around defecation-related issues like diarrhea, tenesmus (the urge to defecate without success), or occasional constipation. The presence of blood or blood-tinged mucus during bowel movements is common among individuals with proctitis.

Proctosigmoiditis: Inflammation extends to both the rectum and the sigmoid colon, the latter being the final segment of the colon adjacent to the rectum. While constipation is rare, symptoms closely mirror those of proctitis. Compared to more extensive colonic involvement, proctosigmoiditis tends to entail fewer health complications.

Colitis of the distal colon: Also known as left-sided colitis, this subtype affects the left side of the colon, including the sigmoid colon and the rectum. It stands as the most prevalent form of UC, prompting recent treatment strategies to focus on medications targeting the distal portion of the colorectal area. In addition to previously mentioned symptoms, distal colitis can induce left-sided abdominal pain.

Pancolitis: This variant, also referred to as total or universal colitis, spans the entire colorectal region.

Severe abdominal pain and cramping, along with recurrent diarrhea episodes often containing blood, mucus, and pus, characterize pancolitis. Nutrient absorption by the colon may be compromised, potentially impacting overall health. Systemic complications such as fever and weight loss might also manifest.

Colitis with severe manifestations: In this form, the majority of the colon is affected, except for the portion directly adjoining the small intestine. Symptoms, treatment, and prognosis closely resemble those of pancolitis.

Fulminant colitis (rare): Representing one of the rarest and most severe forms, fulminant colitis typically affects individuals previously diagnosed with a less severe UC subtype. Symptoms include intense and prolonged diarrhea, severe pain and cramping, and significant bleeding. Immediate medical attention is crucial in cases of fulminant colitis to prevent life-threatening complications like toxic megacolon if left untreated.

What exactly triggers ulcerative colitis?

The precise origins of ulcerative colitis remain shrouded in mystery, yet prevailing theories point to an intricate interplay of factors within the body's immune system. At its core, ulcerative colitis is often classified as an autoimmune disorder, wherein the body's immune defenses mistakenly target healthy tissues, sparking inflammation and a cascade of symptoms.

In the intricate dance of immunity, the immune system stands as the sentinel against invading pathogens. However, in cases of ulcerative colitis, this system misidentifies benign bacteria within the colon as hostile invaders, triggering an inflammatory response that wreaks havoc on the colon and rectum. Alternatively, some researchers propose that a prior viral or bacterial infection might serve as the catalyst, triggering an immune response that fails to abate even after the initial threat has passed, perpetuating a cycle of inflammation.

Furthermore, there are hypotheses suggesting that ulcerative colitis might stem from a malfunction in the immune system itself, or from an imbalance between beneficial and harmful bacteria within the gastrointestinal tract.

Genetics also emerge as a significant player in the development of ulcerative colitis. Evidence suggests that inherited genes can predispose individuals to this condition, with a familial history serving as a potential indicator of susceptibility. Researchers have pinpointed several genes linked to immune system function that may heighten the risk of developing ulcerative colitis, further emphasizing the genetic component of this complex disorder.

Yet, the environment also exerts a profound influence on the onset and progression of ulcerative colitis. Geographical location and lifestyle factors intertwine to shape an individual's risk profile, with higher prevalence observed in certain regions and urban environments. Environmental elements such as air pollution, medication use, and dietary patterns have all been scrutinized for their potential contributions to the disease. Despite ongoing research, no definitive environmental factors have been identified, though regions with improved sanitation exhibit higher rates of ulcerative colitis, hinting at the nuanced relationship between bacterial exposure and disease risk.

Ulcerative colitis emerges as a multifaceted interplay between genetic predisposition, immune dysregulation, and environmental influences. Understanding these complex interactions holds the key to unraveling the mysteries of this debilitating condition and paving the way for more effective treatments and preventative strategies.

SECTION 2: SIGNS AND SYMPTOMS OF ULCERATIVE COLITIS

Living with ulcerative colitis can manifest in a myriad of symptoms, each varying in intensity and impact on one's daily life. These symptoms encompass gastrointestinal issues, such as diarrhea often accompanied by blood, mucus, or pus, along with rectal discomfort, abdominal cramping, and a frequent urge to urinate.

However, the effects of ulcerative colitis extend beyond the digestive tract, influencing overall health and potentially affecting other parts of the body. These extraintestinal manifestations might include involuntary weight loss, decreased appetite, malnutrition, and fatigue, as well as inflammation of the eyes, skin, or joints.

It's important to note that not everyone experiences the full spectrum of potential symptoms associated with ulcerative colitis. Individuals with this condition often observe fluctuations in their symptoms over time, cycling between periods of flare-ups and remission.

During flare-ups, when inflammation is active and new damage to the intestinal tissue occurs, individuals may experience heightened or worsening symptoms. Conversely, remission periods allow the intestinal tissue to heal, with symptoms either absent or sufficiently mild to not significantly interfere with daily activities.

Despite treatment efforts, flare-ups can still occur, with symptoms varying from person to person based on factors such as the type and severity of ulcerative colitis. Frequent or prolonged flare-ups may increase the risk of developing related health complications.

People in remission are typically advised to promptly contact their healthcare provider if they suspect the onset of a flare-up, enabling the development of a tailored treatment plan. Severe flare-ups may present additional symptoms, including breathing difficulties, rapid or irregular heartbeat, and dangerously high temperatures, necessitating immediate medical attention.

How can you tell if you have ulcerative colitis?

Your healthcare provider will conduct a thorough physical examination as part of your medical assessment. This typically involves a series of tests to evaluate your overall health and identify any potential issues. One such test is a blood test, which helps assess the composition of your blood, including the number of red and white blood cells present. Low red blood cell counts may indicate anemia, while elevated white blood cell counts can be a sign of inflammation or infection.

In addition to blood tests, there are other diagnostic procedures commonly used to evaluate conditions like ulcerative colitis. Stool sample analysis is one such method, where a small sample of stool is examined for abnormal bacteria or signs of bleeding or infection. This analysis helps identify potential causes of digestive issues like diarrhea.

Another diagnostic tool is upper endoscopy, also known as EGD (esophagogastroduodenoscopy), which allows for the examination of the esophagus, stomach, and upper part of the small intestine. During this procedure, a flexible, lighted tube with a camera is inserted through the mouth and throat to visualize these organs and take tissue samples if necessary.

Colonoscopy is another common procedure used to assess the health of the large intestine. A long, flexible tube equipped with a camera is inserted through the rectum to examine the colon lining for abnormalities such as growths, inflammation, ulcers, or bleeding. Tissue samples can also be taken during this procedure for further analysis.

Biopsy involves the extraction of tissue samples from the colon lining for microscopic examination. This helps identify any abnormalities or signs of disease.

Additionally, lower gastrointestinal (GI) series, also known as a barium enema, may be performed. This involves coating the rectum, large intestine, and lower small intestine with a metallic fluid called barium, which makes them visible on X-rays. This procedure can help detect strictures, blockages, or other issues within the intestines.

While blood tests alone cannot diagnose or rule out ulcerative colitis, they can provide valuable information for monitoring the disease. These tests, along with other diagnostic procedures, play a crucial role in evaluating and managing ulcerative colitis and other gastrointestinal conditions.

What might my experience be like if doctors diagnose me with ulcerative colitis?

Ulcerative colitis is a chronic condition that can bring about a wide spectrum of symptoms, varying from mild inconveniences to severe disruptions in daily life. For many individuals, these symptoms ebb and flow, coming and going in unpredictable patterns. Some may experience only a single episode before rebounding back to health, while others find themselves grappling with a relentless and swiftly progressing form of the disease.

In up to 30% of cases, ulcerative colitis extends its reach from the rectum to the colon, potentially exacerbating symptoms and complicating management efforts. The impact can be particularly pronounced when both regions are affected, leading to more intense and frequent bouts of discomfort and distress.

While medication can offer some relief and assistance in managing the disease, it's essential to understand that there's currently no definitive "cure" for ulcerative colitis. In cases where the condition becomes unmanageable or significantly impairs quality of life, surgical intervention may be necessary. Approximately 30% of individuals diagnosed with ulcerative colitis ultimately require surgery to remove the colon and rectum, providing a potential pathway to relief and improved long-term outcomes.

How can I safeguard myself against ulcerative colitis?

The medical community finds itself in a puzzling conundrum when it comes to deciphering the root causes of ulcerative colitis, a perplexing condition that wreaks havoc on the digestive system. Despite tireless efforts, experts remain confounded about how to effectively prevent this disease from taking hold. However, amidst this uncertainty, a beacon of hope emerges in the form of nutritional interventions, which hold promise in managing the symptoms of this debilitating condition.

Harnessing the power of dietary adjustments, individuals grappling with ulcerative colitis can potentially find relief from their discomfort. These dietary modifications, though seemingly simple, can wield significant influence over the course of the disease. Recommendations may include steering clear of carbonated beverages, temporarily avoiding high-fiber foods like popcorn, vegetable skins, and nuts during symptomatic periods, increasing fluid intake, opting for smaller and more frequent meals, and diligently maintaining a food diary to pinpoint potential trigger foods.

In cases where nutrient absorption is compromised, healthcare providers may advise the incorporation of nutritional supplements and vitamins to bridge the gap. It's imperative to keep your healthcare provider informed about any complementary or alternative therapies you may be exploring, such as dietary supplements and probiotics, to ensure comprehensive and safe care.

However, the journey of managing ulcerative colitis extends far beyond mere dietary adjustments. It demands a commitment to long-term management, as the condition can exact a toll not only on one's physical well-being but also on their financial resources and emotional resilience, impacting both the individual and their loved ones. If you find yourself grappling with the challenges posed by this disease, don't hesitate to reach out for support. Mental health counselors and both local and online support groups can offer invaluable guidance and solace during trying times.

Moreover, in certain scenarios, healthcare providers may caution against the use of nonsteroidal anti-inflammatory drugs (NSAIDs) such as ibuprofen, naproxen, or similar pain relievers, as these medications have the potential to exacerbate ulcerative colitis symptoms in susceptible individuals. By heeding such advice and maintaining open communication with healthcare professionals, individuals can navigate the complexities of ulcerative colitis with greater clarity and resilience, ultimately paving the way towards enhanced well-being and quality of life.

SECTION 3: WHAT'S THE TREATMENT FOR ULCERATIVE COLITIS?

Your personalized treatment plan will be crafted with careful consideration of various factors, including your specific symptoms, age, overall health, and the severity of your condition. Additionally, your intended family plans, such as pregnancy, will play a crucial role in determining the most suitable course of action.

While ulcerative colitis typically doesn't necessitate a specialized diet, avoiding foods that seem to trigger discomfort in your intestines might help alleviate mild symptoms. However, in more severe cases, medical intervention may be necessary. Here are some potential avenues of treatment:

Medication: Depending on the severity of your symptoms, your healthcare provider may prescribe medications to reduce inflammation and alleviate stomach cramps. Steroids, antibiotics, or drugs that modulate your immune system might be recommended in more serious cases. However, steroids are generally not recommended for long-term use, and alternative medications for ongoing symptom management will be discussed with you.

Hospitalization: In instances of severe symptoms, hospitalization may be required to provide essential nutrients, control diarrhea, and replenish lost fluids, blood, and electrolytes. Depending on your condition, you might receive a special diet, intravenous (IV) feedings, medications, or even surgical intervention.

Surgery: While surgery is not typically the first-line treatment, it may be necessary in certain circumstances. For instance, if you experience heavy bleeding, profound weakness after prolonged illness, colonic perforation, or are at risk for cancer, surgical removal of the colon may be recommended. Surgery options include:

1. Ileostomy and proctocolectomy: This common procedure involves removing the entire colon and rectum, with a small opening (stoma) created in the abdominal wall. The bottom part of the small intestine (ileum) is then connected to this opening, allowing stool to be collected in a drainage bag.

2. Ileoanal anastomosis: In this procedure, the entire colon and diseased rectal lining are removed, while the outer muscles of the rectum remain intact. The ileum is then connected to the anus, forming a pouch to hold stool. This enables relatively normal passage of stool

through the anus, although bowel movements may be more frequent or watery than usual.

If your colon is retained, regular colonoscopies will be necessary due to the increased risk of colon cancer. Ultimately, the most suitable treatment approach will be determined through collaboration between you and your healthcare team, with careful consideration of your individual circumstances and preferences.

What kind of problems can ulcerative colitis cause?

What Are the Possible Complications of Ulcerative Colitis?

Living with ulcerative colitis (UC) entails not only managing the symptoms but also being aware of potential complications that may arise, particularly if the condition is left untreated or if medication instructions are not strictly followed, such as skipping doses. Here are some of the most common complications associated with UC:

1. Rectal bleeding, if left unchecked, can lead to iron deficiency anemia, affecting overall health and energy levels.

2. Intestinal rupture, though rare, is a serious complication of UC that may require immediate medical attention to prevent further complications such as sepsis.

3. Long-term inflammation and damage to the colon can increase the risk of developing colon cancer, underscoring the importance of regular monitoring and screening.

4. Malabsorption of nutrients due to chronic inflammation can result in vitamin and mineral deficiencies, potentially leading to conditions like osteopenia or osteoporosis, which weaken bones and increase the risk of fractures.

5. UC can also trigger inflammation in other parts of the body, including the eyes, skin, and joints, causing additional discomfort and complications.

For individuals who have undergone UC surgery, it's essential to be mindful of potential surgical complications. Discuss any warning signs or concerns with your healthcare provider to ensure prompt evaluation and appropriate management.

In navigating the complexities of ulcerative colitis, proactive management, adherence to medication regimens, regular monitoring, and open communication with healthcare providers are crucial for minimizing the risk of complications and optimizing overall health and well-being.

How often do I need to get a colonoscopy?

If you're experiencing symptoms or undergoing medication adjustments, your doctor might recommend regular examinations of your rectum and colon to ensure that your treatments are effective and your intestinal lining is healing properly. The frequency of these examinations can vary depending on individual circumstances.

Furthermore, individuals with ulcerative colitis are at a higher risk of developing colon cancer. As a precautionary measure, your healthcare provider may schedule you for a colonoscopy every one to three years to screen for any early signs of cancer and monitor the overall health of your colon. This procedure is crucial for early detection and intervention, potentially saving lives through timely treatment.

When should I reach out to a doctor regarding my ulcerative colitis?

If you find yourself experiencing any of the following symptoms, it's essential to reach out to your healthcare provider promptly:

1. Persistent and severe diarrhea: If you notice that your bowel movements have become frequent, watery, and accompanied by abdominal discomfort, it's crucial to seek medical attention. Diarrhea can lead to dehydration and may be a sign of an underlying condition that requires treatment.

2. Presence of blood clots in your stool: Seeing blood in your stool can be alarming, especially if it appears in the form of clots. This could indicate bleeding from the lower gastrointestinal tract, such as the rectum or

colon. It's important not to ignore this symptom, as it may signify serious conditions like hemorrhoids, inflammatory bowel disease, or colorectal cancer.

3. High fever accompanied by persistent pain: A sudden onset of high fever coupled with continuous, unrelenting pain should never be overlooked. These symptoms could be indicative of a severe infection or inflammation within the body, such as appendicitis, diverticulitis, or kidney infection. Prompt medical evaluation is necessary to determine the cause and initiate appropriate treatment.

Remember, your health and well-being are paramount, and seeking timely medical assistance can help ensure that any underlying issues are addressed promptly and effectively. Don't hesitate to reach out to your doctor if you're experiencing any concerning symptoms.

What are some important questions I should ask my child's doctor to ensure I'm advocating for their health effectively?

Apart from the inquiries provided earlier, it's essential to engage your healthcare provider with additional questions pertinent to your child's well-being and specific circumstances:

1. Vitamin Recommendations: Seeking guidance on the appropriate vitamins for your child can ensure their nutritional needs are met. Inquire about the specific supplements or dietary adjustments that may benefit their growth and development.

2.Sibling Concerns: If pediatric ulcerative colitis is diagnosed in one child, it's natural to wonder about the likelihood of it affecting other siblings. Discussing this with your healthcare provider can provide insights into familial predispositions and potential preventive measures.

3.Risk Assessment for Other Conditions: Understanding the broader health implications for your child is crucial. Inquire about any heightened risks for other illnesses or conditions related to pediatric ulcerative colitis, allowing for proactive management strategies to be implemented.

4. Mental Health Support: Dealing with the emotional toll of pediatric ulcerative colitis can be challenging for children. Asking your healthcare provider for

recommendations on mental health professionals such as psychiatrists or therapists can facilitate coping mechanisms and emotional well-being for your child.

5.Developmental Milestones: Monitoring your child's developmental progress is integral to ensuring they are thriving in various aspects of their growth. Inquire about their developmental trajectory to address any concerns or identify areas where additional support may be beneficial.

6. School Adjustment Strategies: Transitioning back to school or adapting to academic environments can pose unique challenges for children managing health conditions. Seek advice from your healthcare provider on effective strategies and accommodations to support your child's adjustment to school life while managing pediatric ulcerative colitis.

By proactively engaging your healthcare provider with these inquiries, you can equip yourself with a comprehensive understanding of your child's health needs and collaborate effectively in their care journey.

SECTION 4: YOUR MENTAL WELL-BEING AND ULCERATIVE COLITIS

Undoubtedly, the impact of ulcerative colitis (UC) on mental health cannot be overstated. The intricate interplay between the mind and the gut means that the everyday pressures of life can materialize as distressing digestive symptoms. This symbiotic relationship is a two-way street: stress can exacerbate gastrointestinal (GI) symptoms, which in turn can amplify stress levels, creating a cyclic pattern of distress.

Moreover, scholarly investigations, such as a recent study highlighted in the Canadian Journal of Gastroenterology and Hepatology, underscore that individuals grappling with inflammatory bowel disease (IBD), including UC, face an elevated risk of experiencing symptoms associated with anxiety and depression. In some cases, these symptoms can progress into clinically significant mood disorders. This correlation isn't surprising when considering the lived experience of navigating a condition like UC, which is often accompanied by societal stigma, leading to feelings of isolation. The persistent apprehension of symptom flare-ups can induce anxiety and stress, disrupting daily activities such as work, school, and social interactions, thereby significantly impacting one's mental well-being.

Establishing a robust support network comprising understanding friends, empathetic family members, and a compassionate healthcare team is paramount in alleviating the emotional toll of UC. Additionally, seeking guidance from a therapist can offer invaluable assistance. Therapists equipped with specialized techniques can empower individuals with UC to manage anxiety effectively, reframe negative thought patterns, and cultivate resilience in the face of adversity. By proactively addressing the intersection of UC and mental health, individuals can embark on a journey towards holistic well-being, fostering a sense of empowerment and control over their health outcomes.

How does pediatric ulcerative colitis affect my child's emotional well-being and mental health?

Ulcerative colitis, much like numerous other ailments, possesses the potential to exert a significant negative psychological toll, especially on the delicate minds of children. Amidst grappling with the physical manifestations of the illness, children often find themselves besieged by a plethora of emotional, social, and familial challenges. The administration of medications coupled with the overarching stress of the situation can catalyze an array of distressing symptoms within your child:

1. Fluctuating Moods: The rollercoaster of emotions becomes a daily reality.

2. Bullying and Teasing: Facing taunts and jeers from classmates adds an extra layer of anguish.

3. Feelings of Anger, Embarrassment, and Frustration: The constant battle against their own bodies can be overwhelmingly disheartening.

4. Self-consciousness Regarding Appearance and Physical Endurance: Concerns about how they look and their ability to keep up physically become a constant source of worry.

5. Vulnerability due to Impaired Bodily Functions: Feeling exposed and vulnerable due to the body's inability to function normally.

6. Difficulty Concentrating: The cognitive fog induced by the illness makes focusing on tasks a Herculean feat.

7. Communication Breakdowns with Friends and Family: Misunderstandings and strained interactions become commonplace.

Navigating through these tumultuous waters necessitates a united front of familial support. It is imperative for the entire family unit to familiarize themselves with the intricacies of the disease and strive to foster an environment of empathy and understanding. Seeking the guidance of both a psychiatrist and a therapist can provide invaluable assistance in equipping your child with the tools necessary to confront and overcome the myriad challenges presented by ulcerative colitis.

What are some good questions to ask my doctor?

If you're grappling with the complexities of ulcerative colitis, it's paramount to schedule a comprehensive consultation with your healthcare provider to delve into the multifaceted considerations surrounding your condition. Here are several pivotal inquiries to embark upon during your discussion:

1. Determining the Extent of Affliction:

It's imperative to discern the precise extent to which your large intestine is affected by this inflammatory bowel disease. Understanding the specific regions impacted can provide crucial insights into crafting an effective treatment plan tailored to your unique circumstances.

2. Unveiling Potential Risks and Side Effects:

Delve into a thorough examination of the potential risks and side effects associated with the medications prescribed to manage your condition. Gaining a comprehensive understanding of these nuances empowers you to make informed decisions regarding your healthcare journey.

3. Navigating Dietary Adjustments:

Explore the possibility of implementing dietary modifications to alleviate symptoms and optimize your overall well-being. Your healthcare provider can offer personalized guidance on dietary adjustments that may complement your treatment regimen and enhance your quality of life.

4. Fertility Concerns and Conception:

If you have aspirations of starting or expanding your family, it's natural to harbor concerns regarding how ulcerative colitis may impact your fertility and ability to conceive. Engage in candid discussions with your healthcare provider to address any apprehensions and explore potential strategies for navigating this aspect of your health journey.

5. Implementing Symptom Management Strategies:

Seek insights into practical measures you can undertake at home to effectively manage and mitigate the symptoms of ulcerative colitis. From lifestyle modifications to self-care practices, understanding how to proactively address symptoms empowers you to maintain a sense of control and well-being amidst the challenges posed by this chronic condition.

6. Exploring Surgical Interventions:

Inquire about the array of surgical options available for managing ulcerative colitis, should conservative treatments prove insufficient in mitigating your symptoms or addressing disease progression. Understanding the potential surgical interventions empowers you to make informed decisions regarding your long-term treatment strategy and overall health trajectory.

By engaging in open, transparent dialogue with your healthcare provider and proactively addressing these critical inquiries, you can navigate the complexities of ulcerative colitis with confidence and forge a path towards optimal health and well-being.

Can Ulcerative Colitis Weaken Your Immune System?

Ulcerative colitis, while not directly impairing your immune system, may prompt alterations in how your immune system functions due to the medications prescribed for its management. It's important to recognize that these alterations can vary depending on the specific medication utilized in treatment. Consequently, certain adjustments may heighten the susceptibility to particular infections or introduce other health concerns.

Engaging in thorough discussions with your healthcare team prior to initiating any medication regimen is paramount. These discussions provide an opportunity to comprehensively understand the potential risks associated with the prescribed medications and devise strategies to mitigate them effectively. By fostering open dialogue with your healthcare providers, you empower yourself to make informed decisions regarding your treatment plan, thereby promoting optimal health outcomes and minimizing potential complications.

SECTION 5: DIET AND MANAGING ULCERATIVE COLITIS?

Ulcerative colitis, a chronic inflammatory bowel disease, isn't solely triggered by dietary factors, nor can it be remedied by any specific dietary regimen. However, the foods one consumes could potentially influence symptom management and the frequency of flare-ups. It's important to recognize that certain foods might exacerbate symptoms and should be avoided, especially during flare-ups. These trigger foods can vary from individual to individual. Keeping a detailed food journal can aid in identifying which specific foods adversely affect you, thereby allowing for a more tailored approach to dietary management.

In particular, individuals with ulcerative colitis are often advised to steer clear of greasy foods, sugary items, carbonated beverages, high-fiber foods, and alcohol. Moreover, infants, children, and teenagers with the condition may encounter difficulties with dairy products and excessive salt intake. Monitoring a child's dietary intake becomes crucial during flare-ups, as reduced appetite and compromised nutrient absorption due to inflammation can impact their growth and overall health. Consequently, it may be necessary to increase caloric intake to ensure adequate nutrition.

For individuals, or caregivers of those with ulcerative colitis, collaborating with healthcare providers and nutritionists is paramount in devising a personalized dietary plan. By working together, they can navigate the complexities of managing the condition through dietary adjustments, ensuring optimal nutrition while minimizing symptom aggravation and flare-ups.

What diet works best for managing ulcerative colitis?

Designing an optimal dietary regimen for managing ulcerative colitis isn't a one-size-fits-all endeavor. The intricate interplay between your unique physiology and the condition's impact on your colon's lining means that standard dietary recommendations might not suffice. Ulcerative colitis can impede the absorption of essential nutrients from food, posing a challenge to maintaining adequate nutrition solely through dietary means.

In such cases, your healthcare provider might suggest incorporating supplemental nutrition or specific vitamins to address potential deficiencies and support your overall well-being. However, determining the most suitable approach requires a personalized touch, taking into account various factors such as your medical history, current health status, medication regimen, and dietary preferences.

Crafting a personalized dietary plan entails a collaborative effort involving not only your healthcare provider but also a qualified nutritionist. By consulting with these professionals, you can gain valuable insights into tailoring your diet to better manage ulcerative colitis while ensuring optimal nutrition intake. Together, you can explore strategies to mitigate symptoms, alleviate discomfort, and promote gastrointestinal health through dietary modifications and targeted supplementation.

Remember, the journey toward optimal health with ulcerative colitis is multifaceted, and finding the right dietary approach is just one piece of the puzzle. Through proactive collaboration with your healthcare team, you can navigate the complexities of managing this chronic condition while striving for improved quality of life and overall well-being.

SECTION 6: ULCERATIVE COLITIS RECIPES

ULCERATIVE COLITIS BREAKFAST RECIPES

Two-minute breakfast smoothie

Items Needed

1 banana

1 tbsp porridge oats

80g soft fruit (whatever you have – strawberries, blueberries, and mango all work well)

150ml milk

1 tsp honey

1 tsp vanilla extract

Directions

STEP 1

Put all the ingredients in a blender and whizz for 1 min until smooth.

STEP 2

Pour the banana oat smoothie into two glasses to serve.

American blueberry pancakes

Items Needed

200g self-raising flour

1 tsp baking powder

1 egg

300ml milk

knob butter

150g pack blueberry

sunflower oil or a little butter for cooking

golden or maple syrup

Directions

STEP 1

Mix together 200g self-raising flour, 1 tsp baking powder and a pinch of salt in a large bowl.

STEP 2

Beat 1 egg with 300ml milk, make a well in the centre of the dry ingredients and whisk in the milk to make a thick smooth batter.

STEP 3

Beat in a knob of melted butter, and gently stir in half of the 150g pack of blueberries.

STEP 4

Heat a teaspoon of sunflower oil or small knob of butter in a large non-stick frying pan.

STEP 5

Drop a large tablespoonful of the batter per pancake into the pan to make pancakes about 7.5cm across. Make three or four pancakes at a time.

STEP 6

Cook for about 3 minutes over a medium heat until small bubbles appear on the surface of each pancake, then turn and cook another 2-3 minutes until golden.

STEP 7

Cover with kitchen paper to keep warm while you use up the rest of the batter.

STEP 8

Serve with golden or maple syrup and the rest of the blueberries.

Apricot & hazelnut muesli

Items Needed

250g porridge oats

75g blanched hazelnuts, halved

75g pumpkin seeds

1 ½ tsp ground cinnamon

75g sulphur-free dried apricots, chopped

20g apple fruit crisps, or dried apple

600ml fortified oat milk

240g blueberries

Directions

STEP 1

Toast the porridge oats in a frying pan over a gentle heat, stirring frequently. Turn off the heat and stir in the nuts, seeds and cinnamon until fully combined.

STEP 2

Tip into a large bowl, stirring to help it cool, then add the fruit, breaking the apple crisps into smaller pieces. Toss to combine.

STEP 3

If you're following our Healthy Diet Plan, tip two-thirds into an airtight container for other days on the plan. Will keep for up to two weeks. Serve the rest in two bowls with 100ml milk and 40g berries in each.

Budget porridge

Items Needed

85g porridge oats

½tsp ground cinnamon, plus extra to serve (optional)

250ml fortified soya milk, plus 4 tbsp to serve

2 small apples, preferably red

15g raisins

7-8 walnut halves, about 15g, broken

Directions

STEP 1

Tip the oats and cinnamon into a non-stick pan with 150ml water and the 250ml soya milk. Put the pan over a gentle heat. Once simmering, leave for 5 mins, stirring frequently (as soya milk has a tendency to stick) until the porridge has thickened.

STEP 2

Meanwhile, coarsely grate the apples, including the skin, into a bowl, until you're just left with the cores.

STEP 3

Serve the porridge with the apple, raisins and nuts on top, and sprinkle over some extra cinnamon, if you like. Stir through the extra soya milk to loosen.

Herb omelette with fried tomatoes

Items Needed

1 tsp olive oil

3 tomatoes, halved

4 large eggs

1 tbsp chopped parsley

1 tbsp chopped basil

Directions

STEP 1

Heat the oil in a small non-stick frying pan, then cook the tomatoes cut-side down until starting to soften and colour. Meanwhile, beat the eggs with the herbs and plenty of freshly ground black pepper in a small bowl.

STEP 2

Scoop the tomatoes from the pan and put them on two serving plates. Pour the egg mixture into the pan and stir gently with a wooden spoon so the egg that sets on the base of the pan moves to enable uncooked egg to flow into the space. Stop stirring when it's nearly cooked to allow it to set into an omelette. Cut into four and serve with the tomatoes.

Basic omelette recipe

Items Needed

3 eggs, beaten

1 tsp sunflower oil

1 tsp butter

Directions

STEP 1

Season the beaten eggs well with salt and pepper. Heat the oil and butter in a non-stick frying pan over a medium-low heat until the butter has melted and is foaming.

STEP 2

Pour the eggs into the pan, tilt the pan ever so slightly from one side to another to allow the eggs to swirl and cover the surface of the pan completely. Let the mixture cook for about 20 seconds then scrape a line through the middle with a spatula.

STEP 3

Tilt the pan again to allow it to fill back up with the runny egg. Repeat once or twice more until the egg has just set.

STEP 4

At this point you can fill the omelette with whatever you like – some grated cheese, sliced ham, fresh herbs, sautéed mushrooms or smoked salmon all work well. Scatter the filling over the top of the omelette and fold gently in half with the spatula. Slide onto a plate to serve.

Easy banana pancakes

Items Needed

350g self-raising flour

1 tsp baking powder

2 very ripe bananas

2 medium eggs

1 tsp vanilla extract

250ml whole milk

butter, for frying

To serve

2 just ripe bananas, sliced

maple syrup (optional)

pecan halves, toasted and roughly chopped (optional)

Directions

STEP 1

Sieve the flour, baking powder and a generous pinch of salt into a large bowl. In a separate mixing bowl, mash the very ripe bananas with a fork until smooth, then whisk in the eggs, vanilla extract and milk. Make a well in the centre of the dry Items Needed, tip in the wet Items Needed and swiftly whisk together to create a smooth, silky batter.

STEP 2

Heat a little knob of butter in a large non-stick pan over a medium heat. Add 2-3 tbsp of the batter to the pan and cook for several minutes, or until small bubbles start appearing on the surface. Flip the pancake over and cook for 1-2 mins on the other side. Repeat with the remaining batter, keeping the pancakes warm in a low oven.

STEP 3

Stack the pancakes on plates and top with the banana slices, a glug of sticky maple syrup and a handful of pecan nuts, if you like.

Peach & orange yogurt pots with ginger oats

Items Needed

4 peaches or nectarines, stoned and diced

1 orange, juiced and zested

120g porridge oats

25g pine nuts

½ tsp ground ginger

1 tsp ground cinnamon

2 tbsp sultanas

4 x 150ml pots bio yogurt

Directions

STEP 1

Put the peaches and orange juice in a small pan. Put the lid on and cook gently for 3-5 mins, depending on their ripeness, until softened. Set aside to cool.

STEP 2

Tip the oats and pine nuts into a pan and heat gently, stirring frequently until they're just starting to toast. Turn off the heat and add the spices, zest and sultanas.

STEP 3

Spoon the peaches and juices into four tumblers and top with the yogurt. Cover and chill until needed. Keep the oat mixture in an airtight container. When ready to serve, top the peaches and yogurt with the oat mixture.

Black bean & barley cakes with poached eggs

Items Needed

2 x 400g cans black beans, drained well

15g porridge oats

2 tsp ground coriander

1 tsp cumin seeds

2 tsp thyme leaves

1 tsp vegetable bouillon powder

5 large eggs

2 spring onions, the white part finely chopped, the green thinly sliced

400g can barley, drained

2-3 tsp rapeseed oil

200g pack cherry tomatoes on the vine

4 tbsp sunflower seeds

Directions

STEP 1

Tip the beans, oats, ground coriander, cumin seeds, thyme and vegetable bouillon powder into a bowl and blitz together with a hand blender to make a rough paste. Stir in 1 egg with the whites of the spring onion and barley. If you're following our Healthy Diet Plan, separate half the mix for another morning and chill.

STEP 2

Heat half the oil in your largest frying pan and fry the other half of the mixture in two big spoonfuls, gently pressed to make flat cakes. After 7 mins, carefully turn over to cook the other side for 4-5 mins.

STEP 3

Meanwhile, poach two eggs in a pan of boiling water for 3-4 mins, and gently fry half of the tomatoes on the vine in a little oil for a few mins to brown slightly. Slide the cakes onto plates and top with the tomatoes, eggs, a scattering of the spring onion greens and half the sun ower seeds. On another morning, repeat steps 2 and 3 with the remaining ingredients.

STEP 4

If you're not following the Healthy Diet Plan and you're serving four, follow steps 2 and 3 with all the ingredients instead of only half.

Bircher muesli with apple & banana

Items Needed

1 eating apple, coarsely grated

50g jumbo porridge oats

25g mixed seeds (such as sunflower, pumpkin, sesame and linseed)

25g mixed nuts (such as Brazils, hazelnuts, almonds, pecans and walnuts), roughly chopped

¼ tsp ground cinnamon

100g full-fat natural bio-yogurt

1 medium banana, sliced

25g organic sultanas

Directions

STEP 1

Put the grated apple in a bowl and add the oats, seeds, half the nuts and the cinnamon. Toss together well. Stir in the yogurt and 100ml cold water, cover and chill for several hours or overnight. Spoon the muesli into two bowls and top with the sliced banana, sultanas and remaining nuts.

Tofu scramble

Items Needed

1 tbsp olive oil

1 small onion, finely sliced

1 large garlic clove, crushed

½ tsp turmeric

1 tsp ground cumin

½ tsp sweet smoked paprika

280g extra firm tofu

100g cherry tomatoes, halved

½ small bunch parsley, chopped

rye bread, to serve, (optional)

Directions

STEP 1

Heat the oil in a frying pan over a medium heat and gently fry the onion for 8 -10 mins or until golden brown and sticky. Stir in the garlic, turmeric, cumin and paprika and cook for 1 min.

STEP 2

Roughly mash the tofu in a bowl using a fork, keeping some pieces chunky. Add to the pan and fry for 3 mins. Raise the heat, then tip in the tomatoes, cooking for 5 mins more or until they begin to soften. Fold the parsley through the mixture. Serve on its own or with toasted rye bread (not gluten-free), if you like.

Mushroom brunch

Items Needed

250g mushrooms

1 garlic clove

1 tbsp olive oil

160g bag kale

4 eggs

Directions

STEP 1

Slice the mushrooms and crush the garlic clove. Heat the olive oil in a large non-stick frying pan, then fry the garlic over a low heat for 1 min. Add the mushrooms and cook until soft. Then, add the kale. If the kale won't all fit in the pan, add half and stir until wilted, then add the rest. Once all the kale is wilted, season.

STEP 2

Now crack in the eggs and keep them cooking gently for 2-3 mins. Then, cover with the lid to for a further 2-3 mins or until the eggs are cooked to your liking. Serve with regular or keto bread for a keto-friendly version.

Fluffy American pancakes

Items Needed

8 slices pancetta, to serve (optional)

sunflower oil and butter, for cooking

blueberries, to serve (optional)

For the pancakes

300g self-raising flour

1 tsp baking powder

1 tbsp caster sugar

2 medium eggs

1 tbsp maple syrup, plus extra to serve

300ml milk

Directions

STEP 1

If serving with pancetta, heat oven to 200C/180C fan/gas 6. Line a baking tray with baking parchment and lay on the pancetta in a single layer. Put another piece of parchment on top, followed by a second baking tray, and bake for 12-15 mins until crisp.

STEP 2

To make the pancakes, get a little helper to weigh out and tip the flour, baking powder and sugar into a large bowl with a small pinch of salt. Crack in the eggs and whisk until smooth. Add the maple syrup and milk while whisking.

STEP 3

Heat a splash of oil and a small knob of butter in a non-stick frying pan until sizzling. Add spoonfuls of batter to make pancakes the size you like, we made 20cm pancakes for a serving size of one per person, or if you are very hungry, two per person. Cook until bubbles start to form on the surface, then flip and cook the other side. Eat straight away or keep warm in a low oven while you cook another batch. Serve pancakes with pancetta or blueberries, drizzled with extra maple syrup.

Healthy porridge bowl

Items Needed

100g frozen raspberries

1 orange, ½ sliced and ½ juiced

150g porridge oats

100ml milk

½ banana, sliced

2 tbsp smooth almond butter

1 tbsp goji berries

1 tbsp chia seeds

Directions

STEP 1

Tip half the raspberries and all of the orange juice in a pan. Simmer until the raspberries soften, about 5 mins.

STEP 2

Meanwhile stir the oats, milk and 450ml water in a pan over a low heat until creamy. Top with the raspberry compote, remaining raspberries, orange slices, banana, almond butter, goji berries and chia seeds.

ULCERATIVE COLITIS BRUNCH RECIPES

Huevos rancheros

Items Needed

2 tbsp olive oil

1 small onion, diced

2 garlic cloves, crushed

400g can red kidney beans, drained and rinsed

1 tsp ground cumin

¼ tsp chilli powder

½ tsp dried oregano

4 eggs

4 small flour tortillas, warmed

1 large tomato, diced

handful pickled jalapeño peppers, roughly chopped

30g cheddar, grated

1 avocado, peeled, de-stoned and diced

1 lime, half juiced, half cut into wedges, to serve

chopped coriander, to serve

Directions

STEP 1

Heat 1 tbsp oil in a large pan. Add the onions with a pinch of salt, and cook until translucent, around 3-4 mins. Add the garlic and cook for a minute more.

STEP 2

Stir in the beans, cumin, chilli powder, oregano, some seasoning and 100ml water. Cook for 5-7 mins, stirring occasionally, or until the beans have softened, then remove from the heat, mash and set aside.

STEP 3

Heat the remaining oil in a large frying pan over a medium-high heat. Crack in the eggs, then reduce the heat to low and cook slowly until the whites are completely firm.

STEP 4

To assemble, spread the beans onto the tortillas, add the tomatoes and jalapeños and sprinkle with cheese. Top with some avocado, a squeeze of lime juice and a fried egg, then scatter with coriander. Serve with the lime wedges on the side.

Ham, mushroom & spinach frittata

Items Needed

1 tsp oil

80g chestnut mushrooms, sliced

50g ham, diced

80g bag spinach

4 medium eggs, beaten

1 tbsp grated cheddar

Directions

STEP 1

Heat the grill to its highest setting. Heat the oil in an ovenproof frying pan over a medium-high heat. Tip in the mushrooms and fry for 2 mins until mostly softened. Stir in the ham and spinach, and cook for 1 min more until the spinach has wilted. Season well with black pepper and a pinch of salt.

STEP 2

Reduce the heat and pour over the eggs. Cook undisturbed for 3 mins until the eggs are mostly set. Sprinkle over the cheese and put under the grill for 2 mins. Serve hot or cold.

Oat & chia porridge with prunes

Items Needed

6 prunes

few pinches ground cinnamon

50g traditional oats

2 tbsp chia seeds

½ tsp vanilla extract

300ml bio yogurt

milk, for diluting (optional)

2 small pears, cored and thickly sliced

2 tsp sunflower or pumpkin seeds (optional)

Directions

STEP 1

The night before, put the prunes in a small pan with the cinnamon. Cover scantily with water and bring to the boil, then simmer for 5 mins. Tip into a bowl and set aside to soak overnight.

STEP 2

Put a kettle full of water on to boil. Tip the oats and chia seeds into a bowl, pour over 300ml boiling water then stir well. Cover and leave to soak overnight too.

STEP 3

The next morning, stir the vanilla and half the yogurt into the oat mixture then dilute to the consistency you like best with a little milk or water if necessary. Spoon into bowls and top with the remaining yogurt, the prunes, pears and seeds, if using, then dust with a little more cinnamon, if you like.

Healthy egg & chips

Items Needed

500g potatoes, diced

2 shallots, sliced

1 tbsp olive oil

2 tsp dried crushed oregano or 1 tsp fresh leaves

200g small mushroom

4 eggs

Directions

STEP 1

Heat oven to 200C/fan 180C/gas 6. Tip the potatoes and shallots into a large, non-stick roasting tin, drizzle with the oil, sprinkle over the oregano, then mix everything together well. Bake for 40-45 mins (or until starting to go brown), add the mushrooms, then cook for a further 10 mins until the potatoes are browned and tender.

STEP 2

Make four gaps in the vegetables and crack an egg into each space. Return to the oven for 3-4 mins or until the eggs are cooked to your liking.

Peanut butter & banana on toast

Items Needed

2 slices granary bread

1 small banana

½ tsp cinnamon

1 tbsp crunchy peanut butter

Directions

STEP 1

Toast bread and slice banana. Layer banana on one slice of toast and dust with cinnamon. Spread the second slice with peanut butter, then sandwich the two together and eat straight away.

Homemade muesli with oats, dates & berries

Items Needed

100g traditional oats

12 pecan nuts, broken into pieces

2 tbsp sunflower seeds

6 pitted medjool dates, snipped into pieces

25g high-fibre puffed wheat

4 x pots bio yogurt

300g mixed berries, such as raspberries, strawberries and blueberries

generous sprinkling of ground cinnamon (optional)

Directions

STEP 1

Tip the oats into a frying pan and heat gently, stirring frequently until they are just starting to toast. Add the pecans and seeds to warm briefly, then tip into a large bowl and toss so they cool quickly.

STEP 2

Add the dates and puffed wheat, mix well until thoroughly combined, then serve topped with the yogurt and fruit, and a sprinkling of cinnamon, if you like.

Three-minute blender banana pancakes

Items Needed

small knob of butter, for frying

1 banana

1 egg

1 heaped tbsp self-raising flour

½ tsp baking powder

chopped strawberries and banana, to serve (optional)

maple syrup, to serve (optional)

Directions

STEP 1

Melt the butter in a non-stick frying pan over a low-medium heat. Meanwhile, add the banana, egg, flour and baking powder to a blender and blitz for 20 seconds.

STEP 2

Pour three little puddles straight from the blender into the frying pan. Cook for 1 min or until the tops start to bubble, then flip with a fork or a fish slice and cook for 20-30 seconds more. Repeat with the rest of the mixture to make three more pancakes.

STEP 3

Serve the pancakes with chopped strawberries or banana and a splash of maple syrup, if you like.

Omelette roll-up

Items Needed

1 large egg

a little rapeseed or olive oil for frying

2 tbsp tomato salsa

about 1 tbsp fresh coriander

Directions

STEP 1

Beat the egg with 1 tbsp water. Heat the oil in a medium non-stick pan. Add the egg and swirl round the base of the pan, as though you are making a pancake, and cook until set. There is no need to turn it.

STEP 2

Carefully tip the pancake onto a board, spread with the salsa, sprinkle with the coriander, then roll it up. It can be eaten warm or cold – you can keep it for 2 days in the fridge.

Chocolate chip pancakes

Items Needed

300g self-raising flour

1 tsp baking powder

3 tbsp caster sugar

2 medium eggs

300ml whole milk

150g milk chocolate chips

butter, for frying

whipped cream or ice cream, to serve (optional)

Directions

STEP 1

Sieve the flour, baking powder and ¼ tsp salt into a large mixing bowl. Add the caster sugar and stir until well combined.

STEP 2

Whisk the eggs and milk together in a jug. Make a well in the centre of the dry Items Needed and pour in the wet Items Needed. Use a whisk to combine everything and create a smooth batter. Fold through most of the chocolate chips.

STEP 3

Heat a small knob of butter in a large non-stick frying pan over a medium heat, swirling it round to coat the pan. Add 2-3 tbsp of the batter to the pan and cook for 1-2 mins, or until bubbles begin to rise to the surface. Flip the pancake over and cook for 2 mins on the other side for the same amount of time, or until golden brown and puffed up. Repeat with the remaining batter, keeping the pancakes warm in a low oven.

STEP 4

Stack the pancakes on plates and top with any leftover chocolate chips and a dollop of whipped cream or ice cream, if you like.

Almond crêpes with avocado & nectarines

Items Needed

2 large eggs

3 tbsp ground almonds

2 tsp rapeseed oil

1 avocado, halved, stoned and flesh lightly crushed

2 ripe nectarines, stoned and sliced

seeds from 1/2 pomegranate

½ lime, cut into 2 wedges, for squeezing over

Directions

STEP 1

Beat one egg and 1 1 /2 tbsp of the almonds in a small bowl with 1 tbsp water. Heat 1 tsp oil in a large non-stick frying pan over a medium heat and pour in the egg mixture, swirling the pan to evenly cover the base. Cook until the mixture sets and turns golden on the underside, about 2 mins. (There is no need to flip it over.) Turn it out onto a plate and make another one with 1 tbsp water, the remaining egg, oil and almonds.

STEP 2

Top each crêpe with the avocado, nectarines and pomegranate, and squeeze over the lime at the table.

Power Pancakes

Items Needed

200g plain flour

½ tbsp baking powder

½ tsp fine salt

50g golden caster sugar

1 large egg, beaten

300ml milk

vegetable oil, for cooking

butter, maple syrup and fruit to serve (optional)

Directions

STEP 1

Sieve the flour into a bowl, and add the baking powder, sugar and ½ tsp of salt. Whisk the egg and milk together in a jug, then pour into the bowl and whisk for a few minutes until you make a smooth thick batter.

STEP 2

Add a drizzle of oil to a hot plate or large frying pan, and spread using a piece of kitchen paper. Heat the pan over a medium heat, and once hot, drop 2 tbsp of the batter into the pan to make small pancakes. You will be able to make about 4-5 at a time.

STEP 3

Cook the pancakes for 2-3 mins until the edges are set, and bubbles rise from the middle. Flip and cook for another 2-3 minutes until golden brown and cooked through. Repeat with the remaining batter, keeping the cooked ones warm in a low oven, if you like. Add another drizzle of oil to the pan when needed.

STEP 4

Top the pancakes with a little butter and a drizzle of maple syrup, alongside some seasonal fruit, if you like.

Homemade soft pretzels

Items Needed

500g strong white bread flour

7g sachet fast-action dried yeast

25g dark brown muscovado sugar

50g unsalted butter, melted

plain flour, for dusting

oil, for greasing

3 tbsp bicarbonate of soda, baked (see below)

1 large egg, lightly beaten, for glazing

flaked sea salt, to serve

Directions

STEP 1

Put the flour, yeast, sugar and 1 tsp salt in a large bowl and mix together to combine. In a large jug, mix together 300ml lukewarm water and the butter. Make a well in the flour mixture and pour in the water, mixing together to form a rough dough.

STEP 2

Tip out onto a floured work surface and knead for 10-15 mins or until smooth and elastic. Put the dough in a lightly oiled bowl, cover with oiled cling film and set aside until doubled in size, about 1hr.

STEP 3

Once risen, knock out the air bubbles in the dough and divide into 8 equal pieces. Using your hands, roll each piece into a long rope about 60cm long.

STEP 4

To form into pretzels, lay the rope in a U-shape with the curve pointing towards you. Take the two ends and cross them over.

STEP 5

Take the ends, lift them backwards and press them into the curve of the U-shape. Repeat with the remaining dough. Heat oven to 200C/180C fan/gas 6.

STEP 6

Carefully place the pretzels on a baking tray lined with parchment and lightly greased with oil. Cover lightly with oiled cling film. Set aside for about 20 mins until puffy (not fully risen like bread dough).

STEP 7

Fill a medium-sized saucepan with water, bring to the boil, add the baked bicarbonate of soda, then reduce the heat to a low simmer. One at a time, carefully lift the pretzels into the pan and cook for 20 secs per side. The pretzels will rise to the surface; flip with a slotted spoon.

STEP 8

Use the spoon to gently lift the pretzels from the pan and return them to the baking tray. Once they have all been cooked in the water, lightly brush with the egg and sprinkle with flaked sea salt.

STEP 9

Bake in the oven for 20-25 mins or until a rich, dark brown. Allow to cool on the baking tray for 10 mins, then transfer to a wire rack to cool completely. Best served on the day made but can be frozen for up to 1 month.

Pink barley porridge with vanilla yogurt

Items Needed

100g pearl barley

75g traditional oats

4 large or 8 small ripe red plums, stoned and chopped

½ tsp vanilla extract

4 x bio yogurt

2 tbsp sunflower seeds

Directions

STEP 1

Tip the barley and oats into a bowl, pour over 1 litre boiling water and stir well. Cover and leave to soak overnight.

STEP 2

The next morning, tip the mixture into a pan and stir in the plums. Simmer for 15 mins, stirring frequently and adding a little water if necessary to get a consistency you like.

STEP 3

Stir the vanilla into the yogurt and serve on top of the porridge with the seeds sprinkled over.

Akoori (Indian scrambled eggs)

Items Needed

1 tbsp butter

1 small red onion, finely chopped

1 green or red chilli, deseeded and finely chopped

2 garlic cloves, crushed

¼ tsp ground cumin

¼ tsp garam masala

good pinch of turmeric

2 large tomatoes, deseeded and finely chopped

7 eggs, beaten

small pack coriander, roughly chopped

4 chapatis (or gluten-free alternative), lightly toasted, to serve

Directions

STEP 1

Heat a large frying pan over a low-medium heat and add the butter. Gently fry the onion, chilli and garlic until the onion is soft – about 5 mins. Add the spices and cook for 1-2 mins more, stirring around the pan until aromatic.

STEP 2

Add the tomatoes, cook for 1 min, then pour in the eggs and lower the heat. Stir slowly to scramble the eggs as they cook, and remove from the heat while they are still a little runny. Continue stirring off the heat for 1 min more until the eggs are just set.

STEP 3

Stir through the coriander and serve with chapatis for a delicious breakfast or brunch.

Fluffy American pancakes with cherry-berry syrup

Items Needed

350g self-raising flour

2 tsp baking powder

¼ tsp ground cinnamon

2 tsp caster sugar, plus 2 tbsp

2 large eggs

150g buttermilk or plain yogurt

325ml milk

200g fresh or frozen blueberries

150g frozen or canned pitted cherries

1 tsp cornflour

1 vanilla pod, or 1 tsp bean paste or extract

200g thick-cut smoked streaky bacon

flavourless oil, such as vegetable or sunflower, for frying

200g mascarpone

maple syrup, to serve

Directions

STEP 1

Make the pancake batter up to a day ahead, or just before cooking. Tip the flour, baking powder, cinnamon and 2 tsp sugar into a bowl, add a good pinch of salt and combine with a whisk. Add the eggs, buttermilk or yogurt and milk to the bowl and whisk into a smooth batter. If making ahead, cover and chill until ready to cook.

STEP 2

Tip the blueberries, cherries, cornflour, 2 tbsp sugar and the vanilla into a pan, and stir until the berries are coated in cornflour. Add 1 tbsp water, then place over a high heat and bubble for a minute or 2 until syrupy but the berries are still holding their shape. Set aside to cool, then remove the vanilla pod, if using. This is best served warm.

STEP 3

Heat the grill to medium-high and arrange the bacon on a baking tray lined with foil. Set aside. If you have a separate oven, heat this to a low setting (50C/30C fan/gas ½) with a baking tray in it (this is to keep the pancakes warm as you cook them). If not, they can sit under the bacon, just keep a close eye on them.

STEP 4

Heat a glug of oil in a large, heavy frying pan, wipe the oil around the pan with a piece of kitchen paper, leaving a fine coating of oil on the surface. Transfer the pancake batter to a jug. When the pan is hot but not smoking (keep it over a moderate heat) pour the batter into the pan, making 7-8cm pancakes, with plenty of space between them (you should fit three pancakes in at a time). The batter should sizzle a little as it hits the pan, but not aggressively –

adjust the heat if you need to. Cook each pancake until the underside is golden; by this time bubbles should be appearing on the surface and the edges beginning to set, indicating that the pancake is ready to flip over. Use a fish slice to do this. They should take roughly 2 mins on each side. Transfer the pancakes to the warm baking tray. Wipe a little more oil around the pan and continue cooking the rest of the batter in this way. You should make 12 pancakes.

STEP 5

When you're halfway through the batter, grill the bacon for 4-5 mins on each side until crispy.

STEP 6

To serve, stack the pancakes with a dollop of mascarpone, bacon, and fruits between each layer, and serve with a jug of maple syrup.

ULCERATIVE COLITIS LUNCH RECIPES

Spiced carrot & lentil soup

Items Needed

2 tsp cumin seeds

pinch chilli flakes

2 tbsp olive oil

600g carrots, washed and coarsely grated (no need to peel)

140g split red lentils

1l hot vegetable stock (from a cube is fine)

125ml milk (to make it dairy-free, see 'try' below)

plain yogurt and naan bread, to serve

Directions

STEP 1

Heat a large saucepan and dry-fry 2 tsp cumin seeds and a pinch of chilli flakes for 1 min, or until they start to jump around the pan and release their aromas.

STEP 2

Scoop out about half with a spoon and set aside. Add 2 tbsp olive oil, 600g coarsely grated carrots, 140g split red lentils, 1l hot vegetable stock and 125ml milk to the pan and bring to the boil.

STEP 3

Simmer for 15 mins until the lentils have swollen and softened.

STEP 4

Whizz the soup with a stick blender or in a food processor until smooth (or leave it chunky if you prefer).

STEP 5

Season to taste and finish with a dollop of plain yogurt and a sprinkling of the reserved toasted spices. Serve with warmed naan breads.

Low-fat Spanish omelette

Items Needed

180g sweet potato, peeled and cut into 2cm chunks

5ml olive oil

55g onion, sliced

140g red pepper, diced

1 garlic clove, grated

5 slices turkey bacon, sliced

1 rosemary sprig (optional)

5 eggs (1 whole egg and 4 egg whites)

2 handfuls green salad leaves

150g 0% fat Greek yogurt

Directions

STEP 1

Heat oven to 180C/160C fan/gas 4. Heat the sweet potato chunks in the microwave for 3 mins, leave to rest for 2 mins, then heat again for a further 2 mins, by which time they should be cooked through and soft.

STEP 2

Meanwhile, heat the oil in a nonstick ovenproof frying pan over a medium-high heat. Add the onion, pepper, turkey, garlic and rosemary (if using), and cook for 2-3 mins. When the potatoes are ready, add them to the pan as well.

STEP 3

Beat the egg and egg whites together, then pour into the frying pan. Use a spatula to move the eggs around, scraping it up from the base, for 1-2 mins or until there is a good proportion of cooked egg in the pan and the ingredients are well mixed. Put the pan in the oven and heat until the egg is cooked through. Slide the omelette from the pan and enjoy with a side salad and a good dollop of yogurt.

Chicken satay salad

Items Needed

1 tbsp tamari

1 tsp medium curry powder

¼ tsp ground cumin

1 garlic clove, finely grated

1 tsp clear honey

2 skinless chicken breast fillets (or use turkey breast)

1 tbsp crunchy peanut butter (choose a sugar-free version with no palm oil, if possible)

1 tbsp sweet chilli sauce

1 tbsp lime juice

sunflower oil, for wiping the pan

2 Little Gem lettuce hearts, cut into wedges

¼ cucumber, halved and sliced

1 banana shallot, halved and thinly sliced

coriander, chopped

seeds from ½ pomegranate

Directions

STEP 1

Pour the tamari into a large dish and stir in the curry powder, cumin, garlic and honey. Mix well. Slice the chicken breasts in half horizontally to make 4 fillets in total, then add to the marinade and mix well to coat. Set aside in the fridge for at least 1 hr, or overnight, to allow the flavours to penetrate the chicken.

STEP 2

Meanwhile, mix the peanut butter with the chilli sauce, lime juice, and 1 tbsp water to make a spoonable sauce. When ready to cook the chicken, wipe a large non-stick frying pan with a little oil. Add the chicken and cook, covered with a lid, for 5-6 mins on a medium heat, turning the fillets over for the last min, until cooked but still moist. Set aside, covered, to rest for a few mins.

STEP 3

While the chicken rests, toss the lettuce wedges with the cucumber, shallot, coriander and pomegranate, and pile onto plates. Spoon over a little sauce. Slice the chicken, pile on top of the salad and spoon over the remaining sauce. Eat while the chicken is still warm.

Spicy chicken & avocado wraps

Items Needed

1 chicken breast (approx 180g), thinly sliced at an angle

generous squeeze juice 0.5 lime

½ tsp mild chilli powder

1 garlic clove, chopped

1 tsp olive oil

2 seeded wraps

1 avocado, halved and stoned

1 roasted red pepper from a jar, sliced

a few sprigs coriander, chopped

Directions

STEP 1

Mix the chicken with the lime juice, chilli powder and garlic.

STEP 2

Heat the oil in a non-stick frying pan then fry the chicken for a couple of mins – it will cook very quickly so keep an eye on it. Meanwhile, warm the wraps following the pack instructions or, if you have a gas hob, heat them over the flame to slightly char them. Do not let them dry out or they are difficult to roll.

STEP 3

Squash half an avocado onto each wrap, add the peppers to the pan to warm them through then pile onto the wraps with the chicken, and sprinkle over the coriander. Roll up, cut in half and eat with your fingers.

Prawn & harissa spaghetti

Items Needed

100g long-stem broccoli, cut into thirds

180g dried spaghetti, regular or wholemeal

2 tbsp olive oil

1 large garlic clove, lightly bashed

150g cherry tomatoes, halved

150g raw king prawns

1 heaped tbsp rose harissa paste

1 lemon, finely zested

Directions

STEP 1

Bring a pan of lightly salted water to the boil. Add the broccoli and boil for 1 min 30 secs, or until tender. Drain and set aside. Cook the pasta following pack instructions, then drain, reserving a ladleful of cooking water.

STEP 2

Heat the oil in a large frying pan, add the garlic clove and fry over a low heat for 2 mins.

Remove with a slotted spoon and discard, leaving the flavoured oil.

STEP 3

Add the tomatoes to the pan and fry over a medium heat for 5 mins, or until beginning to soften and turn juicy. Stir through the prawns and cook for 2 mins, or until turning pink. Add the harissa and lemon zest, stirring to coat.

STEP 4

Toss the cooked spaghetti and pasta water through the prawns and harissa. Stir through the broccoli, season to taste and serve.

Courgette, leek & goat's cheese soup

Items Needed

1 tbsp rapeseed oil

400g leeks, well washed and sliced

450g courgettes, sliced

3 tsp vegetable bouillon powder, made up to 1 litre with boiling water

400g spinach

150g tub soft vegetarian goat's cheese

15g basil, plus a few leaves to serve

8 tsp omega seed mix (see tip)

4 x 25g portions wholegrain rye bread

Directions

STEP 1

Heat the oil in a large pan and fry the leeks for a few mins to soften. Add the courgettes, then cover the pan and cook for 5 mins more. Pour in the stock, cover and cook for about 7 mins.

STEP 2

Add the spinach, then cover the pan and cook for 5 mins so that it wilts. Take off the heat and blitz until really smooth with a hand blender. Add the goat's cheese and basil, then blitz again.

STEP 3

If you're making this recipe as part of our two-person Summer Healthy Diet Plan, spoon half the soup into two bowls or large flasks, then cool and chill the remainder for another day. Reheat in a pan or microwave to serve. If serving in bowls, scatter with some extra basil leaves and the seeds, and eat with the rye bread.

Indian chickpeas with poached eggs

Items Needed

1 tbsp rapeseed oil

2 garlic cloves, chopped

1 yellow pepper, deseeded and diced

½ - 1 red chilli, deseeded and chopped

½ bunch spring onions (about 5), tops and whites sliced but kept separate

1 tsp cumin, plus a little extra to serve (optional)

1 tsp coriander

½ tsp turmeric

3 tomatoes, cut into wedges

⅓ pack coriander, chopped

400g can chickpeas in water, drained but liquid reserved

½ tsp reduced-salt bouillon powder (we used Marigold)

4 large eggs

Directions

STEP 1

Heat the oil in a non-stick sauté pan, add the garlic, pepper, chilli and the whites from the spring onions, and fry for 5 mins over a medium-high heat. Meanwhile, put a large pan of water on to boil.

STEP 2

Add the spices, tomatoes, most of the coriander and the chickpeas to the sauté pan and cook for 1-2 mins more. Stir in the bouillon powder and enough liquid from the chickpeas to moisten everything, and leave to simmer gently.

STEP 3

Once the water is at a rolling boil, crack in your eggs and poach for 2 mins, then remove with a slotted spoon. Stir the spring onion tops into the chickpeas, then very lightly crush a few of the chickpeas with a fork or potato masher. Spoon the chickpea mixture onto plates, scatter with the reserved coriander and top with the eggs. Serve with an extra sprinkle of cumin, if you like.

Quick seafood linguine

Items Needed

1 tbsp olive oil

1 onion, chopped

1 garlic clove, chopped

1 tsp paprika

400g can chopped tomatoes

1l chicken stock (from a cube is fine)

300g linguine or spaghetti, roughly broken

240g frozen seafood mix, defrosted

handful of parsley leaves, chopped, and lemon wedges, to serve

Directions

STEP 1

Heat the oil in a wok or large frying pan, then cook the onion and garlic over a medium heat for 5 mins until soft. Add the paprika, tomatoes and stock, then bring to the boil.

STEP 2

Turn down the heat to a simmer, stir in the pasta and cook for 7 mins, stirring occasionally to stop the pasta from sticking. Stir in the seafood, cook for 3 mins more until it's all heated through and the pasta is cooked, then season to taste. Sprinkle with the parsley and serve with lemon wedges.

Versatile veg soup

Items Needed

200g chopped vegetables such as onions, celery and carrots

300g potatoes, cubed

1 tbsp oil

700ml stock

crème fraîche and fresh herbs, to serve

Directions

STEP 1

Fry the vegetables and potatoes in a pan with the oil for a few minutes until beginning to soften.

STEP 2

Cover with the stock and simmer for 10-15 mins until the veg is tender. Blend until smooth, then season. Serve with a dollop of crème fraîche and some fresh herbs. Will freeze for up to one month.

Falafel burgers

Items Needed

400g can chickpeas, rinsed and drained

1 small red onion, roughly chopped

1 garlic clove, chopped

handful of flat-leaf parsley or curly parsley

1 tsp ground cumin

1 tsp ground coriander

½ tsp harissa paste or chilli powder

2 tbsp plain flour

2 tbsp sunflower oil

toasted pitta bread, to serve

200g tub tomato salsa, to serve

green salad, to serve

Directions

STEP 1

Drain the chickpeas and pat dry with kitchen paper. Tip into a food processor along with the onion, garlic, parsley, cumin, coriander, harissa paste, flour and a little salt. Blend until fairly smooth, then shape into four patties with your hands.

STEP 2

Heat the sunflower oil in a non-stick frying pan, and fry the burgers for 3 mins on each side until lightly golden. Serve with the toasted pitta bread, tomato salsa and green salad.

Meatball & tomato soup

Items Needed

1½ tbsp rapeseed oil

1 onion, finely chopped

2 red peppers, deseeded and sliced

1 garlic clove, crushed

½ tsp chilli flakes

2 x 400g cans chopped tomatoes

100g giant couscous

500ml hot vegetable stock

12 pork meatballs

150g baby spinach

½ small bunch of basil

grated parmesan, to serve (optional)

Directions

STEP 1

Heat the oil in a saucepan. Fry the onion and peppers for 7 mins, then stir through the garlic and chilli flakes and cook for 1 min. Add the tomatoes, giant couscous and veg stock and bring to a simmer.

STEP 2

Season to taste, then add the meatballs and spinach. Simmer for 5-7 mins or until cooked through. Ladle into bowls and top with the basil and some parmesan, if you like.

Cod with cucumber, avocado & mango salsa salad

Items Needed

2 x skinless cod fillets

1 lime, zested and juiced

1 small mango, peeled, stoned and chopped (or 2 peaches, stoned and chopped)

1 small avocado, stoned, peeled and sliced

¼ cucumber, chopped

160g cherry tomatoes, quartered

1 red chilli, deseeded and chopped

2 spring onions, sliced

handful chopped coriander

Directions

STEP 1

Heat oven to 200C/180C fan/gas 6. Put the fish in a shallow ovenproof dish and pour over half the lime juice, with a little of the zest, then grind over some black pepper. Bake for 8 mins or until the fish flakes easily but is still moist.

STEP 2

Meanwhile, put the rest of the ingredients, plus the remaining lime juice and zest, in a bowl and combine well. Spoon onto plates and top with the cod, spooning over any juices in the dish.

Best Yorkshire puddings

Items Needed

140g plain flour (this is about 200ml/7fl oz)

4 eggs (200ml/7fl oz)

200ml milk

sunflower oil, for cooking

Directions

STEP 1

Heat oven to 230C/fan 210C/gas 8.

STEP 2

Drizzle a little sunflower oil evenly into two 4-hole Yorkshire pudding tins or two 12-hole non-stick muffin tins and place in the oven to heat through.

STEP 3

To make the batter, tip 140g plain flour into a bowl and beat in 4 eggs until smooth.

STEP 4

Gradually add 200ml milk and carry on beating until the mix is completely lump-free. Season with salt and pepper.

STEP 5

Pour the batter into a jug, then remove the hot tins from the oven. Carefully and evenly pour the batter into the holes.

STEP 6

Place the tins back in the oven and leave undisturbed for 20-25 mins until the puddings have puffed up and browned.

STEP 7

Serve immediately. You can now cool them and freeze for up to 1 month.

Carrot biryani

Items Needed

2 tbsp olive oil

1 onion, sliced

1 green chilli, chopped (deseeded if you don't like it very hot)

1 garlic clove, peeled

1 tbsp garam masala

1 tsp turmeric

3 carrots, grated

2 x 200g pouch brown basmati rice

150g frozen peas

50g roasted cashews

coriander and yogurt, to serve

Directions

STEP 1

Heat the oil in a large frying pan, tip in the onion with a big pinch of salt and fry until softened, around 5 mins, then add the chilli and crush in the garlic and cook for 1 min more. Stir in the spices with a splash of water and cook for a couple of mins before adding the carrots and stirring well to coat in all of the spices and flavours.

STEP 2

Tip in the rice, peas and cashews, then use the back of your spoon to break up any clumps of rice and combine with the rest of the ingredients, cover and cook over a high heat for 5 mins (it's nice if a bit of rice catches on the base to give a bit of texture to the dish). Scatter over the coriander with spoonfuls of yogurt, then serve straight from the pan.

Red lentil soup

Items Needed

1 white onion, finely sliced

2 tsp olive oil

3 garlic cloves, sliced

2 carrots, scrubbed and diced

85g red lentils

1 vegetable stock cube, crumbled

generous sprigs parsley, chopped (about 2 tbsp) plus a few extra leaves

Directions

STEP 1

Put the kettle on to boil while you finely slice the onion. Heat the oil in a medium pan, add the onion and fry for 2 mins while you slice the garlic and dice the carrots. Add them to the pan, and cook briefly over the heat.

STEP 2

Pour in 1 litre of the boiling water from the kettle, stir in the lentils and stock cube, then cover the pan and cook over a medium heat for 15 mins until the lentils are tender. Take off the heat and stir in the parsley. Ladle into bowls, and scatter with extra parsley leaves, if you like.

Epic summer salad

Items Needed

400g black beans, drained

2 large handfuls baby spinach leaves, roughly chopped

500g heritage tomatoes, chopped into large chunks

½ cucumber, halved lengthways, seeds scooped out and sliced on an angle

1 mango, peeled and chopped into chunks

1 large red onion, halved and finely sliced

6-8 radishes, sliced

2 avocados, peeled and sliced

100g feta, crumbled

handful of herbs (reserved from the dressing)

For the dressing

large bunch mint

small bunch coriander

small bunch basil

1 fat green chilli, deseeded and chopped

1 small garlic clove

100ml extra virgin olive oil or rapeseed oil

2 limes, zested and juiced

2 tbsp white wine vinegar

2 tsp honey

Directions

STEP 1

Make the dressing by blending all of the ingredients in a food processor (or very finely chop them), saving a few herb leaves for the salad. You can make the dressing up to 24 hrs before serving.

STEP 2

Scatter the beans and spinach over a large platter. Arrange the tomatoes, cucumber, mango, onion and radishes on top and gently toss together with your hands. Top the salad with the avocados, feta and herbs, and serve the dressing on the side.

Vegetarian fajitas

Items Needed

400g can black beans, drained

small bunch coriander, finely chopped

4 large or 8-12 small flour tortillas

1 avocado, sliced, or 1 small tub guacamole

2 tbsp soured cream or crème fraîche

For the fajita mix

1 red and 1 yellow pepper, cut into strips

1 tbsp oil

1 red onion, cut into thin wedges

1 garlic clove, crushed

½ tsp chilli powder

½ tsp smoked paprika

½ tsp ground cumin

1 lime, juiced

Directions

STEP 1

To make the fajita mix, take two or three strips from each colour of pepper and finely chop them. Set aside. Heat the oil in a frying pan and fry the remaining pepper strips and the onion until soft and starting to brown at the edges. Cool slightly and mix in the chopped raw peppers. Add the garlic and cook for 1 min, then add the spices and stir. Cook for a couple of mins more until the spices become aromatic, then add half the lime juice and season. Transfer to a dish, leaving any juices behind, and keep warm.

STEP 2

Tip the black beans into the same pan, then add the remaining lime juice and plenty of seasoning. Stir the beans around the pan to warm them through and help them absorb any flavours of the fajita mix, then stir through the coriander.

STEP 3

Warm the tortillas in a microwave or in a low oven, then wrap them so they don't dry out. Serve the tortillas with the fajita mix, beans, avocado and soured cream for everyone to help themselves.

Nutty chicken satay strips

Items Needed

2 tbsp chunky peanut butter (without palm oil or sugar)

1 garlic clove, finely grated

1 tsp Madras curry powder

few shakes soy sauce

2 tsp lime juice

2 skinless, chicken breast fillets (about 300g)
cut into thick strips

about 10cm cucumber, cut into fingers

sweet chilli sauce, to serve

Directions

STEP 1

Heat oven to 200C/180C fan/gas 4 and line a
baking tray with non-stick paper.

STEP 2

Mix 2 tbsp chunky peanut butter with 1 finely grated garlic clove, 1 tsp Madras curry powder, a few shakes of soy sauce and 2 tsp lime juice in a bowl. Some nut butters are thicker than others, so if necessary, add a dash of boiling water to get a coating consistency.

STEP 3

Add 2 skinless chicken breast fillets, cut into strips, and mix well. Arrange on the baking sheet, spaced apart, and bake in the oven for 8-10 mins until cooked, but still juicy.

STEP 4

Eat warm with roughly 10cm cucumber, cut into fingers, and sweet chilli sauce.

Alternatively, leave to cool and keep in the fridge for up to 2 days.

Spiced halloumi & pineapple burger with zingy slaw

Items Needed

½ red cabbage, grated

2 carrots, grated

100g radishes, sliced

1 small pack coriander, chopped

2 limes, juiced

1 tbsp cold-pressed rapeseed oil

big pinch of chilli flakes

1 tbsp chipotle paste

60g halloumi, cut into 4 slices

2 small slices of fresh pineapple

1 Little Gem lettuce, divided into 4 lettuce cups, or 2 small seeded burger buns, cut in half, to serve (optional)

Directions

STEP 1

Heat the barbecue. Put the cabbage, carrot, radish and coriander in a bowl. Pour over the lime juice, add ½ tbsp oil and the chilli flakes, then season with salt and pepper. Give everything a good mix with your hands. This can be done a few hours before and kept in the fridge.

STEP 2

Mix the remaining oil with the chipotle paste then coat the halloumi slices in the mixture. Put the halloumi slices on a sheet of foil and put on the barbecue with the pineapple (or use a searing hot griddle pan if cooking inside). Cook for 2 mins on each side until the cheese is golden, and the pineapple is beginning to caramelise. Brush the buns with the remaining chipotle oil, then put your burger buns, if using, cut-side down, on the barbecue for the last 30 seconds of cooking to toast.

STEP 3

Assemble your burgers with the lettuce or buns. Start with a handful of the slaw, then add halloumi and pineapple. Serve with the remaining slaw.

Creamy spinach & mushroom penne

Items Needed

175g wholemeal penne

50g unroasted, unsalted cashews

10g dried porcini mushrooms

1 tsp vegetable bouillon powder

1 tbsp rapeseed oil

120g chestnut mushrooms, halved if large, thinly sliced

2 large garlic cloves, finely grated

200g baby spinach

Directions

STEP 1

Cook the penne following pack instructions and put the kettle on to boil. Meanwhile, put the cashews and dried mushrooms in a medium heatproof bowl along with the bouillon powder, and pour over 200ml boiling water from the kettle. Leave to soak for 5 mins. After this time, blitz the mixture with a hand blender until smooth and creamy.

STEP 2

Heat the oil in a large non-stick frying pan over a medium heat and fry the fresh mushrooms and garlic for a couple of minutes until just starting to soften. Add the spinach and continue to cook, stirring frequently until the spinach has wilted. Drain the pasta, reserving a little of the cooking water. Tip the pasta into the pan with the mushroom mixture, season with plenty of black pepper and toss everything together well. Remove from the heat and stir through the creamy mushroom sauce, adding a drop of the reserved cooking water if needed to loosen. Serve straightaway.

ULCERATIVE COLITIS DINNER RECIPES

Low-fat moussaka

Items Needed

200g frozen sliced peppers

3 garlic cloves, crushed

200g extra-lean minced beef

100g red lentils

2 tsp dried oregano, plus extra for sprinkling

500ml carton passata

1 aubergine, sliced into 1.5cm rounds

4 tomatoes, sliced into 1cm rounds

2 tsp olive oil

25g parmesan, finely grated

170g pot 0% fat Greek yogurt

freshly grated nutmeg

Directions

STEP 1

Cook the peppers gently in a large non-stick pan for about 5 mins – the water from them should stop them sticking. Add the garlic and cook for 1 min more, then add the beef, breaking up with a fork, and cook until brown. Tip in the lentils, half the oregano, the passata and a splash of water. Simmer for 15-20 mins until the lentils are tender, adding more water if you need to.

STEP 2

Meanwhile, heat the grill to Medium. Arrange the aubergine and tomato slices on a non-stick baking tray and brush with the oil. Sprinkle with the remaining oregano and some seasoning, then grill for 1-2 mins each side until lightly charred – you may need to do this in batches.

STEP 3

Mix half the Parmesan with the yogurt and some seasoning. Divide the beef mixture between 4 small ovenproof dishes and top with the sliced aubergine and tomato. Spoon over the yogurt topping and sprinkle with the extra oregano, Parmesan and nutmeg. Grill for 3-4 mins until bubbling. Serve with a salad, if you like.

Burnt aubergine veggie chilli

Items Needed

1 aubergine

1 tbsp olive oil or rapeseed oil

1 red onion, diced

2 carrots, finely diced

70g puy lentils or green lentils, rinsed

30g red lentils, rinsed

400g can kidney beans

3 tbsp dark soy sauce

400g can chopped tomatoes

20g dark chocolate, finely chopped

¼ tsp chilli powder

2 tsp dried oregano

2 tsp ground cumin

2 tsp sweet smoked paprika

1 tsp coriander

1 tsp cinnamon

800ml vegetable stock

½ lime, juiced

To serve

brown rice

tortilla chips, mashed avocado, yogurt or soured cream, grated cheddar, roughly chopped coriander (optional)

Directions

STEP 1

If you have a gas hob, put the aubergine directly onto a lit ring to char completely, turning occasionally with kitchen tongs, until burnt all over. Alternatively, use a barbecue or heat the grill to its highest setting and cook, turning occasionally, until completely blackened (the grill won't give you the same smoky flavour).

Set aside to cool on a plate, then peel off the charred skin and remove the stem. Roughly chop the flesh and set aside.

STEP 2

In a large pan, heat the oil, add the onion and carrots with a pinch of salt, and fry over a low-medium heat for 15-20 mins until the carrots have softened.

STEP 3

Add the aubergine, both types of lentils, the kidney beans with the liquid from the can, soy sauce, tomatoes, chocolate, chilli powder, oregano and the spices. Stir to combine, then pour in the stock. Bring to the boil, then turn down the heat to very low. Cover with a lid and cook for 1½ hrs, checking and stirring every 15-20 mins to prevent it from burning.

STEP 4

Remove the lid and let the mixture simmer over a low-medium heat, stirring occasionally, for about 15 mins until you get a thick sauce. Stir in the lime juice and taste for seasoning – add more salt if needed. Serve hot over rice with whichever accompaniments you want!

Easy sausage casserole

Items Needed

2 tbsp olive or rapeseed oil

1 onion, finely chopped

2 medium sticks celery, finely chopped

1 yellow pepper, chopped

1 red pepper, chopped

6 cooking chorizo sausages (about 400g)

6 pork sausages (about 400g)

3 fat garlic cloves, chopped

1 ½ tsp sweet smoked paprika

½ tsp ground cumin

1 tbsp dried thyme

125ml white wine

2 x 400g cans cherry tomatoes or chopped tomatoes

2 sprigs fresh thyme

1 chicken stock cube

1 x 400g can aduki beans, drained and rinsed

1 bunch chives, snipped (optional)

Directions

STEP 1

Heat 2 tbsp olive or rapeseed oil in a large heavy-based pan.

STEP 2

Add 1 finely chopped onion and cook gently for 5 minutes.

STEP 3

Add 2 finely chopped medium celery sticks, 1 chopped yellow pepper and 1 chopped red pepper and cook for a further 5 mins.

STEP 4

Add 6 chorizo sausages and 6 pork sausages and fry for 5 minutes.

STEP 5

Stir in 3 chopped garlic cloves, 1 ½ tsp sweet smoked paprika, ½ tsp ground cumin and 1 tbsp dried thyme and continue cooking for 1 – 2 mins or until the aromas are released.

STEP 6

Pour in 125ml white wine and use a wooden spoon to remove any residue stuck to the pan.

STEP 7

Add two 400g cans of tomatoes, and 2 sprigs of fresh thyme and bring to a simmer. Crumble in the chicken stock cube and stir.

STEP 8

Cook for 40 minutes. Stir in a 400g drained and rinsed can of aduki beans and cook for a further five minutes.

STEP 9

Remove the thyme sprigs, season with black pepper and stir through some snipped chives, if using. Serve.

Spinach, sweet potato & lentil dhal

Items Needed

1 tbsp sesame oil

1 red onion, finely chopped

1 garlic clove, crushed

thumb-sized piece ginger, peeled and finely chopped

1 red chilli, finely chopped

1½ tsp ground turmeric

1½ tsp ground cumin

2 sweet potatoes (about 400g/14oz), cut into even chunks

250g red split lentils

600ml vegetable stock

80g bag of spinach

4 spring onions, sliced on the diagonal, to serve

½ small pack of Thai basil, leaves torn, to serve

Directions

STEP 1

Heat 1 tbsp sesame oil in a wide-based pan with a tight-fitting lid.

STEP 2

Add 1 finely chopped red onion and cook over a low heat for 10 mins, stirring occasionally, until softened.

STEP 3

Add 1 crushed garlic clove, a finely chopped thumb-sized piece of ginger and 1 finely chopped red chilli, cook for 1 min, then add 1½ tsp ground turmeric and 1½ tsp ground cumin and cook for 1 min more.

STEP 4

Turn up the heat to medium, add 2 sweet potatoes, cut into even chunks, and stir everything together so the potato is coated in the spice mixture.

STEP 5

Tip in 250g red split lentils, 600ml vegetable stock and some seasoning.

STEP 6

Bring the liquid to the boil, then reduce the heat, cover and cook for 20 mins until the lentils are tender and the potato is just holding its shape.

STEP 7

Taste and adjust the seasoning, then gently stir in the 80g spinach. Once wilted, top with the 4 diagonally sliced spring onions and ½ small pack torn basil leaves to serve.

STEP 8

Alternatively, allow to cool completely, then divide between airtight containers and store in the fridge for a healthy lunchbox.

Double bean & roasted pepper chilli

Items Needed

2 onions, chopped

2 celery sticks, finely chopped

2 yellow or orange peppers, finely chopped

2 tbsp sunflower oil or rapeseed oil

2 x 460g jars roasted red peppers

2 tsp chipotle paste

2 tbsp red wine vinegar

1 tbsp cocoa powder

1 tbsp dried oregano

1 tbsp sweet smoked paprika

2 tbsp ground cumin

1 tsp ground cinnamon

2 x 400g cans chopped tomatoes

400g can refried beans

3 x 400g cans kidney beans, drained and rinsed

2 x 400g cans black beans, drained and rinsed

Directions

STEP 1

Put the onions, celery and chopped peppers with the oil in your largest flameproof casserole dish or heavy-based saucepan, and fry gently over a low heat until soft but not coloured.

STEP 2

Drain both jars of peppers over a bowl to catch the juices. Put a quarter of the peppers into a food processor with the chipotle paste, vinegar, cocoa, dried spices and herbs. Whizz to a purée, then stir into the softened veg and cook for a few mins.

STEP 3

Add the tomatoes and refried beans with 1 can water and the reserved pepper juice. Simmer for 1 hr until thickened, smoky and the tomato chunks have broken down to a smoother sauce.

STEP 4

At this stage you can cool and chill the sauce if making ahead. Otherwise add the kidney and black beans, and the remaining roasted peppers, cut into bite-sized pieces, then reheat. (This makes a large batch, so once the sauce is ready it might be easier to split it between two pans when you add the beans and peppers.) Once bubbling and the beans are hot, season to taste and serve.

Chinese chicken curry

Items Needed

4 skinless chicken breasts, cut into chunks (or use thighs or drumsticks)

2 tsp cornflour

1 onion, diced

2 tbsp rapeseed oil

1 garlic clove, crushed

2 tsp curry powder

1 tsp turmeric

½ tsp ground ginger

pinch sugar

400ml chicken stock

1 tsp soy sauce

handful frozen peas

rice to serve

Directions

STEP 1

Toss the chicken pieces in the cornflour and season well. Set them aside.

STEP 2

Fry the onion in half of the oil in a wok on a low to medium heat, until it softens – about 5-6 minutes – then add the garlic and cook for a minute. Stir in the spices and sugar and cook for another minute, then add the stock and soy sauce, bring to a simmer and cook for 20 minutes. Tip everything into a blender and blitz until smooth.

STEP 3

Wipe out the pan and fry the chicken in the remaining oil until it is browned all over. Tip the sauce back into the pan and bring everything to a simmer, stir in the peas and cook for 5 minutes. Add a little water if you need to thin the sauce. Serve with rice.

Chicken cacciatore one-pot with orzo

Items Needed

2 tbsp olive oil

4-6 skin-on, bone-in chicken thighs

1 onion, finely sliced

2 garlic cloves, sliced

250ml red wine

2 bay leaves

4 thyme sprigs

2 rosemary sprigs

small bunch of parsley, stalks and leaves separated, finely chopped

2 x 400g cans cherry tomatoes

1 chicken stock cube

1 tbsp balsamic vinegar

2 tbsp capers (optional)

handful of pitted green olives

300g orzo, rinsed (to keep it from getting too sticky when baked)

Directions

STEP 1

Heat the oven to 220C/200C fan/gas 7. Rub 1 tbsp oil over the chicken and season well, then put skin-side up in an ovenproof casserole dish or roasting tin and bake for 20-25 mins until crisp and golden, but not cooked all the way though. Remove from the dish and put on a plate.

STEP 2

Add the remaining oil to the dish, mixing it with the chicken fat. Tip in the onion and garlic, then bake for 5-8 mins until the onion is tender.

STEP 3

Pour in the wine, stirring it with the onions, then leave to evaporate slightly in the residual heat before adding the bay, thyme, rosemary, parsley stalks and tomatoes. Dissolve the stock cube in 300ml boiling water and pour this in, then add the vinegar, capers, if using, olives and orzo. Stir well and season.

STEP 4

Nestle the chicken back in the pan, skin-side up, and roast for 20 mins until the sauce is thickened, the orzo is tender and the meat is cooked through. Give it a stir, then leave for 10 mins for the orzo to absorb the excess liquid. Scatter over the parsley leaves to serve.

Creamy courgette & bacon pasta

Items Needed

1 tsp olive oil

150g diced pancetta or smoked bacon lardons

4 courgettes, coarsely grated

1 garlic clove, crushed

handful freshly grated parmesan

1 small tub (200g) low-fat crème fraîche

300g tagliatelle

Directions

STEP 1

Heat the olive oil in a large frying pan and sizzle the pancetta or bacon for about 5 mins until starting to crisp. Turn up the heat and add the grated courgette to the pan. Cook for 5 mins or until soft and starting to brown then add the garlic and cook for a minute longer. Season and set aside.

STEP 2

Cook the tagliatelle according to the pack instructions and scoop out a cupful of cooking water. Drain the tagliatelle and tip into the frying pan with the bacon and courgette. Over a low heat toss everything together with the crème fraiche and half the Parmesan adding a splash of pasta water too if you need to loosen the sauce. Season to taste and serve twirled into bowls with the remaining Parmesan scattered over.

Meatball & tomato soup

Items Needed

1½ tbsp rapeseed oil

1 onion, finely chopped

2 red peppers, deseeded and sliced

1 garlic clove, crushed

½ tsp chilli flakes

2 x 400g cans chopped tomatoes

100g giant couscous

500ml hot vegetable stock

12 pork meatballs

150g baby spinach

½ small bunch of basil

grated parmesan, to serve (optional)

Directions

STEP 1

Heat the oil in a saucepan. Fry the onion and peppers for 7 mins, then stir through the garlic and chilli flakes and cook for 1 min. Add the tomatoes, giant couscous and veg stock and bring to a simmer.

STEP 2

Season to taste, then add the meatballs and spinach. Simmer for 5-7 mins or until cooked through. Ladle into bowls and top with the basil and some parmesan, if you like.

Chicken & bacon pasta

Items Needed

2 tbsp olive oil

1 tbsp butter

1 onion, finely chopped

1 large garlic clove, finely grated

200ml double cream

100g mascarpone

75g parmesan, finely grated

1 chicken stock cube

2 cooked chicken breasts (about 210g), shredded

8 rashers cooked streaky bacon (about 25g), roughly chopped

300g tagliatelle

¼ small bunch of parsley, finely chopped

green salad, to serve

Directions

STEP 1

Heat the oil and butter in a medium saucepan over a low heat and fry the onion for 10 mins, or until softened and translucent. Add the garlic and cook for 2 mins more. Add the cream, mascarpone, parmesan and stock cube. Give it a stir and add the cooked chicken and bacon to heat through.

STEP 2

Meanwhile, cook the pasta following pack instructions. Reserve 100ml of the pasta water. Toss the pasta in the creamy sauce and enough of the reserved water to loosen. Season with black pepper. Top with the parsley and serve with a green salad.

Prawn tikka masala

Items Needed

1 large onion, roughly chopped

1 thumb-sized piece ginger, peeled and grated

2 large garlic cloves

1 tbsp rapeseed oil

2-3 tbsp tikka curry paste

400g can chopped tomatoes

2 tbsp tomato purée

½ tbsp light brown soft sugar

3 cardamom pods, bashed

200g brown basmati rice

3 tbsp ground almonds

300g raw king prawns

1 tbsp double cream

½ bunch of coriander, roughly chopped

naan breads, warmed, to serve (optional)

Directions

STEP 1

Put the onion, ginger and garlic in a food processor and blitz to a smooth paste. Heat the oil in a large flameproof casserole dish or pan over a medium heat. Add the onion paste and fry for 8 mins or until lightly golden. Stir in the curry paste and fry for 1 min more. Add the tomatoes, tomato purée, sugar and cardamom pods. Bring to a simmer and cook, covered, for another 10 mins.

STEP 2

Cook the rice following pack instructions.

STEP 3

Scoop the cardamom out of the curry sauce and discard, then blitz with a hand blender, or in a clean food processor. Return to the pan, add the almonds and prawns, and cook for 5 mins. Season to taste and stir through the cream and coriander. Serve with the rice and naan breads, if you like.

Sardine pasta with crunchy parsley crumbs

Items Needed

1 tbsp olive oil

50g dried breadcrumbs

3 garlic cloves, finely chopped

1 rosemary sprig, leaves finely chopped

2 x 120g cans sardines, drained

500g passata

50g sliced black olives, drained

350g linguine or fusilli

small pack parsley, leaves chopped

25g parmesan, finely grated

Directions

STEP 1

Heat 1 tsp olive oil in a non-stick frying pan over a low-medium heat. Add the breadcrumbs and cook, stirring, until they start to turn golden. Add another 1 tsp oil and the garlic. Cook, stirring, for a moment, then tip onto a plate and set aside to cool.

STEP 2

Put a large pan of salted water on to boil. Return the frying pan to a medium heat. Add the remaining 1 tsp olive oil with the rosemary and the sardines. Cook for 2-3 mins, gently breaking up the sardines with a wooden spoon.

Pour in the passata, add the olives and leave to simmer gently for about 10 mins.

STEP 3

Meanwhile, add the pasta to the boiling water and cook following pack instructions. Stir the parsley and half the Parmesan into the breadcrumbs. Drain the pasta, reserving a little of the cooking water. Add a splash of the water to the tomato sauce until it is thin enough to coat the pasta, then stir in the remaining Parmesan. Toss the pasta in the sauce and serve in bowls, each topped with a handful of the crunchy breadcrumbs.

Best Yorkshire puddings

Items Needed

140g plain flour (this is about 200ml/7fl oz)

4 eggs (200ml/7fl oz)

200ml milk

sunflower oil, for cooking

Directions

STEP 1

Heat oven to 230C/fan 210C/gas 8.

STEP 2

Drizzle a little sunflower oil evenly into two 4-hole Yorkshire pudding tins or two 12-hole non-stick muffin tins and place in the oven to heat through.

STEP 3

To make the batter, tip 140g plain flour into a bowl and beat in 4 eggs until smooth.

STEP 4

Gradually add 200ml milk and carry on beating until the mix is completely lump-free. Season with salt and pepper.

STEP 5

Pour the batter into a jug, then remove the hot tins from the oven. Carefully and evenly pour the batter into the holes.

STEP 6

Place the tins back in the oven and leave undisturbed for 20-25 mins until the puddings have puffed up and browned.

STEP 7

Serve immediately. You can now cool them and freeze for up to 1 month.

Creamy mushroom pasta

Items Needed

2 tbsp olive oil

1 tbsp butter

1 onion, finely chopped

250g button chestnut mushroom, sliced

1 garlic clove, finely grated

100ml dry white wine

200ml double cream

1 lemon, zest only

200g parmesan (or vegetarian alternative), grated, plus extra to serve

300g tagliatelle or linguini

½ small bunch parsley, finely chopped

Directions

STEP 1

Heat the oil and butter in a medium saucepan. Fry the onion over a low heat for 10 mins or until softened and translucent.

STEP 2

Add the mushrooms and cook for 10 mins over a medium heat. Add the garlic and cook for 2 mins. Add the wine and bring to a simmer, reduce the liquid by half.

STEP 3

Add the double cream and bring to a simmer, then add the lemon zest and parmesan. Season with salt and plenty of black pepper.

STEP 4

Meanwhile, cook the pasta following pack instructions. Reserve 100ml of the pasta water.

Toss the pasta in the pan with the creamy sauce and enough of the reserved water to loosen. Stir through the parsley, divide into bowls and top with extra cheese, if you like.

Courgette, potato & cheddar soup

Items Needed

500g potato, unpeeled and roughly chopped

2 vegetable stock cubes

1kg courgettes, roughly chopped

bunch spring onion, sliced - save 1 for serving, if eating straight away

100g extra-mature cheddar or vegetarian alternative, grated, plus a little extra to serve

good grating fresh nutmeg, plus extra to serve

Directions

STEP 1

Put the potatoes in a large pan with just enough water to cover them and crumble in the stock cubes. Bring to the boil, then cover and cook for 5 mins. Add the courgettes, put the lid back on and cook for 5 mins more. Throw in the spring onions, cover and cook for a final 5 mins.

STEP 2

Take off the heat, then stir in the cheese and season with the nutmeg, salt and pepper. Whizz to a thick soup, adding more hot water until you get the consistency you like. Serve scattered with extra grated cheddar, spring onions and nutmeg or pepper. Or cool and freeze in freezer bags or containers with good lids for up to 3 months.

Chicken and mushrooms

Items Needed

2 tbsp olive oil

500g boneless, skinless chicken thigh

flour, for dusting

50g cubetti di pancetta

300g small button mushroom

2 large shallots, chopped

250ml chicken stock

1 tbsp white wine vinegar

50g frozen pea

small handful parsley, finely chopped

Directions

STEP 1

Heat 1 tbsp oil in a frying pan. Season and dust the chicken with flour, brown on all sides. Remove. Fry the pancetta and mushrooms until softened, then remove.

STEP 2

Add the final tbsp oil and cook shallots for 5 mins. Add the stock and vinegar, bubble for 1-2 mins. Return the chicken, pancetta and mushrooms and cook for 15 mins. Add the peas and parsley and cook for 2 mins more, then serve.

Mushroom risotto

Items Needed

50g dried porcini mushrooms

1 vegetable stock cube

2 tbsp olive oil

1 onion, finely chopped

2 garlic cloves, finely chopped

250g pack chestnut mushrooms, chopped

300g risotto rice, such as arborio

1 x 175ml glass white wine

25g butter

handful parsley leaves, chopped

50g parmesan or Grana Padano, freshly grated

Directions

STEP 1

Put 50g dried porcini mushrooms into a large bowl and pour over 1 litre boiling water. Soak for 20 mins, then drain into a bowl, discarding the last few tbsp of liquid left in the bowl.

STEP 2

Crumble 1 vegetable stock cube into the mushroom liquid, then squeeze the mushrooms gently to remove any liquid.

STEP 3

Heat 2 tbsp olive oil in a shallow saucepan or deep frying pan over a medium flame. Add 1 finely chopped onion and 2 finely chopped garlic cloves, then fry for about 5 mins until soft.

STEP 4

Stir in 250g chopped chestnut mushrooms and the dried mushrooms, season with salt and pepper and continue to cook for 8 mins until the fresh mushrooms have softened.

STEP 5

Tip 300g risotto rice into the pan and cook for 1 min. Pour over a 175ml glass of white wine and let it bubble to nothing so the alcohol evaporates.

STEP 6

Keep the pan over a medium heat and pour in a quarter of the mushroom stock. Simmer the rice, stirring often, until the rice has absorbed all the liquid.

STEP 7

Add about the same amount of stock again and continue to simmer and stir - it should start to become creamy, plump and tender. By the time the final quarter of stock is added, the rice should be almost cooked.

STEP 8

Continue stirring until the rice is cooked. If the rice is still undercooked, add a splash of water. Take the pan off the heat, add 25g butter and scatter over 25g grated parmesan or Grana Padano cheese and half a handful of chopped parsley leaves.

STEP 9

Cover and leave for a few mins so that the rice can take up any excess liquid as it cools a bit. Give the risotto a final stir, spoon into bowls and scatter with the remaining 25g grated cheese and the remaining chopped parsley leaves.

Steamed trout with mint & dill dressing

Items Needed

120g new potatoes, halved

170g pack asparagus spears, woody ends trimmed

1 ½ tsp vegetable bouillon powder made up to 225ml with water

80g fine green beans, trimmed

80g frozen peas

2 skinless trout fillets

2 slices lemon

For the dressing

4 tbsp bio yogurt

1 tsp cider vinegar

¼ tsp English mustard powder

1 tsp finely chopped mint

2 tsp chopped dill

Directions

STEP 1

Put the new potatoes on to simmer in a pan of boiling water until tender. Cut the asparagus in half to shorten the spears and slice the ends without the tips. Tip the bouillon into a wide non-stick pan. Add the asparagus and beans, then cover and cook for 5 mins.

STEP 2

Add the peas to the pan, then top with the trout and lemon slices. Cover again and cook for 5 mins more until the fish flakes really easily, but is still juicy.

STEP 3

Meanwhile, mix the yogurt with the vinegar, mustard powder, mint and dill. Stir in 2-3 tbsp of the fish cooking juices. Put the veg and any remaining pan juices in bowls, top with the fish and herb dressing, then serve with the potatoes.

Linguine with avocado, tomato & lime

Items Needed

115g wholemeal linguine

1 lime, zested and juiced

1 avocado, stoned, peeled, and chopped

2 large ripe tomatoes, chopped

½ pack fresh coriander, chopped

1 red onion, finely chopped

1 red chilli, deseeded and finely chopped (optional)

Directions

STEP 1

Cook the pasta according to pack instructions – about 10 mins. Meanwhile, put the lime juice and zest in a medium bowl with the avocado, tomatoes, coriander, onion and chilli, if using, and mix well.

STEP 2

Drain the pasta, toss into the bowl and mix well. Serve straight away while still warm, or cold.

Pasta alla vodka

Items Needed

2 tbsp olive oil

1 banana shallot or ½ onion, finely chopped

3 garlic cloves, crushed

¼ tsp chilli flakes

100g tomato purée

5 tbsp vodka

100ml double cream

200g penne or rigatoni pasta

30g grated parmesan or vegetarian alternative, plus extra to serve

small handful of basil leaves, to serve

Directions

STEP 1

Heat the oil in a large frying pan or casserole dish. Add the shallot and a large pinch of salt and gently fry over a low heat for 10 mins or until softened and translucent. Add the garlic and chilli flakes and cook for 30 seconds. Stir through the tomato purée, cook for 2 mins, then stir through the vodka and cook for 3 mins. Quickly stir through the cream to combine, then remove from the heat.

STEP 2

Cook the pasta in salted water following pack instructions. Drain and reserve 150ml cooking water. Add roughly 50ml of the water to the tomato sauce, then tip in the pasta and cheese, tossing everything together over a low heat until well coated and glossy (loosen with a splash more of the cooking water if it's a little dry). Season to taste, then serve with a sprinkling of the extra parmesan, a good grinding of black pepper and the basil leaves scattered over the top.

ULCERATIVE COLITIS SOUP RECIPES

One-pot Chinese chicken noodle soup

Items Needed

1 tbsp honey

3 tbsp dark soy

1 red chilli, sliced

1l chicken stock

80g leftover roast chicken (optional)

20g pickled pink ginger or normal ginger, peeled and finely sliced

½ Chinese cabbage, shredded

300g pouch straight-to-wok thick noodles

4 spring onions, sliced

Directions

STEP 1

Drizzle the honey over the base of a large saucepan and bubble briefly to a caramel, then splash in the soy, bubble, add half the chilli and the chicken stock and simmer for 5 mins.

STEP 2

Add the chicken, if using, and ginger, and simmer for another 5 mins. Stir in the cabbage and noodles and cook until just wilted and the noodles have heated through. Ladle into bowls and sprinkle over the remaining chilli and the spring onions.

Herby broccoli & pea soup

Items Needed

1 tbsp rapeseed oil

1 onion, finely chopped

1 large garlic clove, crushed

400g broccoli, chopped into small florets

300g frozen peas

200g chard, chopped

1l low-salt veg stock

½ small bunch of basil, chopped

small bunch of dill, chopped

1 lemon, zested and juiced

2 tbsp pumpkin seeds, toasted

Directions

STEP 1

Heat the oil in a large saucepan. Add the onion and fry for 8 mins until soft and translucent. Add the garlic and cook for 1 min more. Tip in the broccoli, peas and chard, then pour over the stock and bring the mixture to the boil. Reduce the heat to a simmer, cover and cook for 25 mins.

STEP 2

Stir through the herbs, lemon zest and juice, then blitz the soup with a stick blender until completely smooth. Ladle into bowls and serve with the toasted pumpkin seeds scattered over the top.

Warming chicken noodle soup

Items Needed

4 boneless skinless chicken breasts

60ml sake (if you don't have sake, use vodka)

thumb-sized piece ginger, peeled and sliced into matchsticks

3 spring onions, finely sliced on the diagonal, and white and green parts separated

150ml soy sauce

4 tsp sesame oil

2 garlic cloves, grated

600g thick white noodles (such as udon)

2 large long red Serrano chillies, seeds left in and sliced on the diagonal

1 large egg, beaten

small pack coriander

2 tbsp toasted sesame seeds

seaweed flakes, to serve (optional)

Directions

STEP 1

Slice the chicken breasts into strips about 1cm wide and the full length of the breast. Briefly marinate the chicken in the sake and leave to one side for a few mins.

STEP 2

Mix the ginger with the whites of the spring onions, soy sauce, sesame oil and garlic.

STEP 3

Put 2 litres of water in a saucepan and bring to the boil. Pour in the ginger soy mixture, reduce the heat and cook just below a simmer for 5 mins.

STEP 4

Add the chicken and sake mix, noodles and chillies to the stock and turn the heat up. As soon as the broth comes to the boil, turn off the heat. Slowly pour the egg into the broth, stirring all the time. Add the green parts of the spring onions and stir through. Leave to sit for 2 mins.

STEP 5

Ladle the soup evenly into six bowls. Sprinkle with the toasted sesame seeds and coriander, with a few seaweed flakes, if you like.

Soup maker pea & ham soup

Items Needed

1 onion, chopped

1 medium potato, peeled and diced

1litre ham or pork stock

500g frozen petit pois

300g thickly sliced ham, trimmed of any fat and diced

Directions

STEP 1

Put the onion, potatoes, stock and peas into a soup blender, and press the 'smooth soup' function. Make sure you don't fill the soup maker above the max fill line.

STEP 2

Once the cycle is complete, season, and stir in the ham before serving.

Creamy seafood stew

Items Needed

1 tbsp olive oil

1 onion, chopped

2 celery sticks, chopped

1 garlic clove, crushed

175ml white wine

300ml chicken stock

1 tbsp cornflour, mixed to a paste with 1 tbsp cold water

400g bag frozen seafood mix, defrosted

small bunch dill, chopped

5 tbsp half-fat crème fraîche

garlic bread, to serve

Directions

STEP 1

Heat the oil in a large frying pan and cook the onion and celery until soft but not coloured, about 10 mins. Throw in the garlic and cook for 1 min more. Pour in the wine and simmer on a high heat until most has disappeared.

STEP 2

Pour in the stock and cornflour mix and simmer for 5-10 mins, stirring often until thickened. Season, then add the seafood and most of the dill. Simmer for a few mins until piping hot, then stir in the crème fraîche.

STEP 3

Meanwhile, cook the garlic bread following pack instructions. Divide the stew into warm bowls and scatter with the remaining dill. Serve with garlic bread for dipping into the stew.

Leek & butter bean soup with crispy kale & bacon

Items Needed

4 tsp olive oil

500g leeks, sliced

4 thyme sprigs, leaves picked

2 x 400g cans butter beans

500ml vegetable bouillon stock

2 tsp wholegrain mustard

½ small pack flat-leaf parsley

3 rashers streaky bacon

40g chopped kale, any tough stems removed

25g hazelnuts, roughly chopped

Directions

STEP 1

Heat 1 tbsp oil in a large saucepan over a low heat. Add the leeks, thyme and seasoning. Cover and cook for 15 mins until softened, adding a splash of water if the leeks start to stick. Add the butter beans with the water from the cans, the stock and mustard. Bring to the boil and simmer for 3-4 mins until hot. Blend the soup in a food processor or with a stick blender, stir through the parsley and check the seasoning.

STEP 2

Put the bacon in a large, non-stick frying pan over a medium heat. Cook for 3-4 mins until crispy, then set side to cool. Add the remaining 1 tsp oil to the pan, and tip in the kale and hazelnuts. Cook for 2 mins, stirring until the kale is wilted and crisping at the edges and the hazelnuts are toasted. Cut the bacon into small pieces, then stir into the kale mixture.

STEP 3

Reheat the soup, adding a splash of water if it is too thick. Serve in bowls sprinkled with the bacon & kale mixture.

Creamy smoked salmon, leek & potato soup

Items Needed

large knob of butter

2 large leeks, halved and finely sliced

1 bay leaf

1kg floury potatoes, diced

1l chicken or vegetable stock

100ml double cream

200g smoked salmon, cut into strips

small bunch chives, snipped

Directions

STEP 1

Heat the butter in a large saucepan and add the leeks and bay leaf. Cook over a low heat for 8-10 mins or until the leek is really soft, then stir through the potatoes until coated in the butter. Pour over the stock and cream and bring to the simmer, then gently bubble for 10-15 mins until the potatoes are really tender. If freezing at this stage, slightly under-cook the potatoes, then defrost and bring back to a simmer to finish cooking them and continue the recipe.

STEP 2

Add two-thirds of the smoked salmon, stir through and season. Serve the soup in deep bowls with the remaining smoked salmon and snipped chives on the top.

Easy soup maker lentil soup

Items Needed

750ml vegetable or ham stock

75g red lentils

3 carrots, finely chopped

1 medium leek, sliced (150g)

small handful chopped parsley, to serve

Directions

STEP 1

Put the stock, lentils, carrots and leek into a soup maker, and press the 'chunky soup' function. Make sure you don't fill it above the max fill line. The soup will look a little foamy to start, but don't worry – it will disappear once cooked.

STEP 2

Once the cycle is complete, check the lentils are tender, and season well. Scatter over the parsley to serve.

Creamy leek & bean soup

Items Needed

1 tbsp rapeseed oil

600g leeks, well washed and thinly sliced

1l hot vegetable bouillon

2 x 400g cans cannellini beans, drained

2 large garlic cloves, finely grated

100g baby spinach

150ml full-fat milk

Directions

STEP 1

Heat the oil in a large pan, add the leeks and cook on a low-medium heat for 5 mins. Pour in the bouillon, tip in the beans, cover and simmer for 10 mins.

STEP 2

Stir in the garlic and spinach, cover the pan and cook for 5 mins more until the spinach has wilted but still retains its fresh green colour.

STEP 3

Add the milk and plenty of pepper, and blitz with a stick blender until smooth. Ladle into bowls and chill the remainder

Soup maker tomato soup

Items Needed

500g ripe tomatoes, off the vine and quartered or halved

1 small onion, chopped

½ small carrot, chopped

½ celery stick, chopped

1 tsp tomato purée

pinch of sugar

450ml vegetable stock

Directions

STEP 1

Put all the ingredients into the soup maker and press the 'smooth soup' function. Make sure you don't fill the soup maker above the max fill line.

STEP 2

Once the cycle is complete, season well, and check the soup for sweetness. Add a little more sugar, salt or tomato puree for depth of colour, if you like.

Easy soup maker roast chicken soup

Items Needed

1 onion, chopped

1 large carrot, chopped

½ tbsp thyme leaves, roughly chopped

700ml chicken stock

100g frozen peas

150g leftover roast chicken, shredded and skin removed

1½ tbsp Greek yogurt

½ small garlic clove, crushed

squeeze lemon juice

Directions

STEP 1

Put the onion, carrot, thyme, stock, and peas into a soup maker, and press the 'chunky soup' function. Make sure you don't fill the soup maker above the max fill line.

STEP 2

Once the cycle is complete, stir in the shredded roast chicken, and leave to warm through while you mix the yogurt, garlic and lemon juice together. Season the soup, and pour into bowls. Stir in some of the yogurt and serve.

Summer carrot, tarragon & white bean soup

Items Needed

1 tbsp rapeseed oil

2 large leeks, well washed, halved lengthways and finely sliced

700g carrots, chopped

1.4l hot reduced-salt vegetable bouillon (we used Marigold)

4 garlic cloves, finely grated

2 x 400g cans cannellini beans in water

⅔ small pack tarragon, leaves roughly chopped

Directions

STEP 1

Heat the oil over a medium heat in a large pan and fry the leeks and carrots for 5 mins to soften.

STEP 2

Pour over the stock, stir in the garlic, the beans with their liquid, and three-quarters of the tarragon, then cover and simmer for 15 mins or until the veg is just tender. Stir in the remaining tarragon before serving.

Asparagus soup

Items Needed

25g butter

a little vegetable oil

350g asparagus spear, stalks chopped, woody ends discarded, tips reserved

3 shallots, finely sliced

2 garlic cloves, crushed

2 large handfuls spinach

700ml vegetable stock (fresh if possible)

olive oil, for drizzling (optional)

rustic bread (preferably sourdough), to serve (optional)

Directions

STEP 1

Heat the butter and oil in a large saucepan until foaming. Fry the asparagus tips for a few mins to soften. Remove and set aside.

STEP 2

Add the shallots, asparagus stalks and garlic, and cook for 5-10 mins until softened but still bright. Stir through the spinach, pour over the stock, bring to the boil, then blitz with a hand blender.

STEP 3

Season generously and add hot water to loosen if needed. Ladle into bowls and scatter the asparagus tips over each. Drizzle with olive oil and serve with sourdough bread, if you like.

Indian chickpea & vegetable soup

Items Needed

1 tbsp vegetable oil

1 large onion, chopped

1 tsp finely grated fresh root ginger

1 garlic clove, chopped

1 tbsp garam masala

850ml vegetable stock

2 large carrots, quartered lengthways and chopped

400g can chickpea, drained

100g green bean, chopped

Directions

STEP 1

Heat the oil in a medium saucepan, then add the onion, ginger and garlic. Fry for 2 mins, then add the garam masala, give it 1 min more, then add the stock and carrots. Simmer for 10 mins, then add the chickpeas. Use a stick blender to whizz the soup a little. Stir in the beans and simmer for 3 mins. Pack into a flask or, if you've got a microwave at work, chill and heat up for lunch. Great with naan bread.

Smoky tomato, chipotle & charred corn soup

Items Needed

1 tbsp rapeseed oil

1 onion, finely chopped

2 garlic cloves, chopped

2 tsp ground coriander

small bunch of coriander, stalks chopped and leaves left whole

400g can chopped tomatoes

600ml vegetable stock

1-1½ tbsp chipotle chilli paste

2 corn on the cobs

50g feta, crumbled

4 tbsp fat-free Greek yogurt

Directions

STEP 1

Heat the oil in a casserole dish and fry the onion for 10 mins until beginning to soften. Add the garlic, ground coriander and coriander stalks, and cook for 1 min. Stir though the tomatoes, stock and chipotle and bring to a simmer. Cook, covered, over a low heat for 20 mins, stirring occasionally.

STEP 2

Meanwhile, bring a pan of water to the boil and cook the corn for 4 mins. Drain and leave to cool a little. Cut the kernels off the cob with a sharp knife. Heat a non-stick frying pan over a high heat. Add the corn and fry for 5-7 mins or until charred, stirring now and again.

STEP 3

Ladle the soup into bowls. Top with the feta, yogurt, charred corn and coriander leaves.

ULCERATIVE COLITIS -TEAS, SMOOTHIES, AND LATTES

Low-sugar lime & basil green juice

Items Needed

70ml chilled apple and elderflower juice

50g baby spinach

20g basil leaves

6cm piece of cucumber (about 100g), chopped

1 lime, zested and juiced

Directions

STEP 1

Pour the apple juice into a large jug then add the spinach, basil, cucumber, lime and 100ml chilled water.

STEP 2

Blitz really well with a hand blender until very smooth. Pour into a glass and drink straightaway.

Strawberry smoothie

Items Needed

10 strawberries, hulled (approx 175g)

1 small banana, sliced

100ml orange juice, chilled

Directions

STEP 1

Blitz the strawberries in a blender with the banana and orange juice until smooth.

STEP 2

Pour the smoothie into a tall glass to serve.

Strawberry green goddess smoothie

Items Needed

160g ripe strawberries, hulled

160g baby spinach

1 small avocado, halved and the flesh scooped out

150ml pot bio yogurt

2 small oranges, juiced, plus ½ tsp finely grated zest

Directions

STEP 1

Put all the ingredients in a blender and whizz until completely smooth. If it's a little thick, add a drop of chilled water then blitz again. Pour into glasses and drink straight away.

Avocado & strawberry smoothie

Items Needed

½ avocado, stoned, peeled and cut into chunks

150g strawberry, halved

4 tbsp low-fat natural yogurt

200ml semi-skimmed milk

lemon or lime juice, to taste

honey, to taste

Directions

STEP 1

Put all the ingredients in a blender and whizz until smooth. If the consistency is too thick, add a little water.

Turmeric latte

Items Needed

350ml almond milk (or any milk of your choice)

¼ tsp ground turmeric

¼ tsp ground cinnamon

¼ tsp ground ginger

½ tsp vanilla extract

1 tsp maple syrup

grind of black pepper

Directions

STEP 1

Put all the ingredients in a saucepan and whisk constantly over a gentle heat, ideally with a milk frother if you have one. Once hot, pour into mugs and sprinkle with a little more cinnamon to serve.

Gingerbread hot chocolate

Items Needed

150ml milk

50ml double cream

¼-½ tsp dark brown soft sugar

½ orange, zested

pinch of ground ginger

pinch of ground cinnamon

1 clove

2 drops of vanilla extract

50g dark chocolate, chopped

To garnish (optional)

whipped cream

1 mini gingerbread or speculoos biscuit, crushed

Directions

STEP 1

Stir the milk, cream, sugar, orange zest and spices together in a saucepan, then bring to a simmer over a low heat. Remove from the heat and pour through a sieve into a jug, discarding the clove and orange zest. Pour the warm infused milk back into the pan and stir in the vanilla and chocolate until the chocolate has melted and is smooth.

STEP 2

Return the pan to a low heat to warm through, if needed, then pour into a heatproof mug. Top with whipped cream and crushed gingerbread biscuits, if you like, then serve.

Aperol spritz

Items Needed

ice

100ml Aperol

150ml prosecco

soda, to top up

Directions

STEP 1

Put a couple of cubes of ice into 2 glasses and add a 50 ml measure of Aperol to each. Divide the prosecco between the glasses and then top up with soda, if you like.

Sunshine smoothie

Items Needed

500ml carrot juice, chilled

200g pineapple (fresh or canned)

2 bananas, broken into chunks

small piece ginger, peeled

20g cashew nuts

juice 1 lime

Directions

STEP 1

Put the ingredients in a blender and whizz until smooth. Drink straight away or pour into a bottle to drink on the go. Will keep in the fridge for a day.

Iced coffee

Items Needed

200ml strong black coffee

50ml milk

ice

maple syrup, optional

Directions

STEP 1

Make a 200ml cup of black coffee following pack instructions, then allow the coffee to go completely cold. Pour into a blender with the milk along with 2 or 3 handfuls of ice and maple syrup, if using, then blend until smooth and foamy.

STEP 2

Pour into a chilled tall glass and serve.

Pumpkin spice latte

Items Needed

2 tsp pumpkin purée

pinch of ground cinnamon, plus extra to serve (or use pumpkin spice)

pinch of ground ginger

pinch of ground nutmeg

30ml espresso or strong coffee

250ml milk (any will work)

Directions

STEP 1

Put the pumpkin purée in a large heatproof glass or mug. Stir in the spices and espresso or strong coffee.

STEP 2

Heat the milk in a saucepan over a low heat until steaming and frothy. Pour into the glass or mug, and spoon over any froth. Stir to combine, then dust with more cinnamon or some pumpkin spice before serving.

Kiwi fruit smoothie

Items Needed

3 peeled kiwi fruit

1 mango, peeled, stoned and chopped

500ml pineapple juice

1 banana, sliced

Directions

STEP 1

Put all of the ingredients in a blender and blitz until smooth then pour into 2 tall glasses.

Chai tea

Items Needed

2 mugs milk (or use almond milk)

2 English Breakfast tea bags

6 cracked cardamom pods

½ cinnamon stick

a grating of fresh nutmeg

2 cloves

2-4 tsp light brown soft sugar

Directions

STEP 1

Heat the milk in a saucepan over a very low heat. Empty the contents of the tea bags into the pan, then add the cracked cardamom pods, cinnamon stick, nutmeg and cloves.

STEP 2

Sweeten with light brown soft sugar to taste (chai tea should be sweet, but use less if you like), then leave to infuse, but not boil, for 10 mins. Strain into mugs and enjoy.

Rhubarb cordial

Items Needed

300g golden caster sugar

zest and juice 1 orange

zest and juice 1 lemon

450g rhubarb, chopped

1 slice fresh root ginger, peeled

Directions

STEP 1

Put the sugar in a large saucepan with 300ml water. Bring to a simmer then add the zest and juice of both the orange and the lemon along with the rhubarb and the ginger.

STEP 2

Cook the mixture over a medium heat until the rhubarb is falling apart.

STEP 3

Pour the mixture through a sieve lined with muslin into a clean heatproof jug then transfer to sterilised bottles. Keeps in the fridge for up to 1 month.

STEP 4

Serve approx. 25ml of cordial per 100ml sparkling water, or to taste.

Honey and lemon tea

Items Needed

2-3 tsp honey

¼ lemon, juiced, plus 1 slice

Directions

STEP 1

Mix the honey and lemon juice in the bottom of a cup while you boil the kettle. Pour over the hot water, add the lemon slice and stir well to combine. Add another teaspoon of honey if you prefer it sweeter.

Masala chai

Items Needed

200ml-250ml milk (dairy or other)

1-2 tbsp sugar or syrup, like stevia, maple syrup, to taste

For the infusion

3 green cardamom pods, bashed and husks removed

½ cinnamon stick

2 cloves

3 black peppercorns

½ tsp ground ginger

2 tsp loose leaf black tea leaves, such as Assam

Directions

STEP 1

For the infusion, put the cardamom seeds in a pestle and mortar, along with the cinnamon, cloves and peppercorns, and bash to release the oils – you don't want to make a powder. Tip into a pan and stir in the ginger and black tea leaves.

STEP 2

Pour in 400ml water and bring to a very gentle simmer over a low heat, to allow the tea to infuse before it starts to boil. Stir in the milk and sugar or syrup to taste, and remove from the heat. Leave to infuse for 2 mins before straining into mugs.

SECTION 7: ONE MORE THING BEFORE YOU GO!

As we conclude our exploration of ulcerative colitis, it's essential to reflect on the profound impact this condition has on individuals, families, and communities. Beyond its physical manifestations, ulcerative colitis often exacts a toll on emotional well-being, social interactions, and overall quality of life. Through the personal stories shared within these pages, we've witnessed the resilience, courage, and perseverance of those living with this chronic illness.

For many, the journey with ulcerative colitis is marked by a relentless quest for understanding, acceptance, and effective management strategies. It's a journey fraught with challenges, setbacks, and moments of profound vulnerability. Yet, amid the struggles, there are also triumphs, moments of resilience, and acts of profound compassion that illuminate the path forward.

Throughout this book, we've delved into the complexities of ulcerative colitis, exploring its underlying mechanisms, clinical manifestations, and diverse treatment options. We've celebrated the strides made in medical research and innovation while acknowledging the gaps that remain in our understanding and therapeutic approaches.

But perhaps most importantly, we've recognized the power of community, empathy, and support in navigating the uncertainties of life with ulcerative colitis. Whether it's the unwavering support of loved ones, the guidance of compassionate healthcare providers, or the solidarity found in support groups and online forums, no one faces this journey alone.

As we turn the final page, let us carry forward the lessons learned, the bonds forged, and the hope kindled within these chapters. Let us continue to advocate for greater awareness, research, and resources for those affected by ulcerative colitis. And let us never lose sight of the humanity, strength, and resilience that unite us in our shared quest for health, understanding, and compassion. For in the end, it's our collective journey that defines us, empowers us, and inspires us to embrace life's challenges with courage, grace, and unwavering determination.

A Note from the Writer

Ensuring optimal management and care for ulcerative colitis, a chronic inflammatory bowel disease, entails a multifaceted approach that emphasizes the indispensable role of collaboration between patients and their healthcare teams. This partnership serves as the cornerstone for navigating the complexities of the condition, transcending mere symptom management to encompass holistic well-being and disease control.

Central to this collaborative effort is the imperative for patients to remain actively engaged in their treatment journey, regardless of the presence or absence of symptoms. Adherence to prescribed medication regimens stands paramount, as it not only serves to mitigate symptoms but also plays a pivotal role in preventing disease exacerbations. Skipping medications, even during periods of remission, can precipitate flare-ups, compromising the efficacy of treatment and rendering the condition more challenging to manage in the long term.

Moreover, consistent and open communication between patients and their healthcare providers forms the linchpin of effective ulcerative colitis management. Regular dialogues enable healthcare professionals to gain insights into the patient's unique experiences, symptomatology, and treatment response, thereby facilitating informed decision-making and personalized care interventions. Through such ongoing exchanges, patients can actively participate in the formulation of treatment plans tailored to their specific needs, preferences, and lifestyle considerations.

Furthermore, the collaborative approach extends beyond the realm of treatment adherence and encompasses proactive disease monitoring and self-management strategies. Patients are encouraged to remain vigilant for any subtle changes in symptoms or overall health status and to promptly communicate such observations to their healthcare providers. This proactive stance not only fosters early intervention but also empowers patients to take an active role in their health management, thereby enhancing their sense of control and well-being.

The effective management of ulcerative colitis hinges upon the synergistic partnership between patients and their healthcare teams. By embracing a collaborative ethos, characterized by medication adherence, open communication, and proactive self-management, individuals with ulcerative colitis can empower themselves with the knowledge, resources, and support necessary to navigate the challenges posed by this chronic condition and optimize their overall quality of life.